FINALLY
LOSE IT

FINALLY
LOSE IT

A professional woman's guide to
stop dieting, fix your hormones
and overcome weight loss resistance

DR. SARAH WILSON, BSc, ND

DR. SARAH WILSON, ND

ISBN-13: 978-1-7752471-0-4

Edited by Paula Sarson
Cover design © 2018 Valerie Bellamy
Book design and layout by Dog-ear Book Design
Illustrations by Elise Walmsley
Icon designs © dreamstale.com

This book is intended as a reference resource only, not as a medical manual. The information provided in this book is designed to help you make informed decisions about your health. It is not intended to substitute for any medical treatment that may have been prescribed by your medical doctor. If you suspect that you have a medical problem, please seek the advice of a practicing physician. Information provided in this document and your use of any products or services related to this document does not create a doctor-patient relationship between you and Sarah Wilson, ND. This information is not intended to diagnose or treat; therefore, you should contact your medical provider before beginning any new health regime.

The patient cases referenced in this book are provided for the sole purpose of education. Names and personal details have been changed to protect patients' privacy.

To my current and future patients and to my twelve-year-old self:
you are not destined to be overweight, and you can feel well in your body.
This is for you!

Introduction 1

PART ONE

The Finally Lose It Education Plan
Metabolism 101

1   Why Diets Fail 15

2   Find Your Rhythm 23

3   Sleep Your Way Slimmer 49

4   The Truth about Stress and Your Waistline 69

5   It's Called Belly Fat for a Reason
Digestive Hormones and Weight Loss Resistance 101

6   The Fat-Burning Blocker
Insulin and Insulin Resistance 139

7   Get Your Head in the Game 169

TABLE OF CONTENTS

PART TWO
The Finally Lose It Action Plan

8 Let's Talk about Food..187

9 30-Day Start-Up Guide...213

PART THREE
Recipes for Success

10 Recipes...227

APPENDICES

Appendix A
Laboratory testing optimal ranges 275

Appendix B
At-Home Testing 276

References 279

List of Figures...286

Index 287

Acknowledgements 292

About the Author..293

TABLE OF CONTENTS

INTRODUCTION

You are trying to lose weight. You have followed every diet, eaten weird food, and perhaps even taken pills on your desperate quest to finally attain the body you want. Yet, you haven't been able to achieve your weight loss goals. This is called *weight loss resistance*. The concept is a mystery to many, but to me it was life, and my journey to solve this struggle led to my discovery of the principles in this book. It turns out, weight loss resistance is *completely* explainable. I have overcome it for myself and have supported my patients to do the same in my naturopathic medical practice. Now I am sharing these principles with you.

This book is for women, like yourself, who feel as though their doctors are missing something. It is for the women who do all the "right" things—eat a little, exercise a lot, and push themselves to be better—while getting no results. This book will educate you about what causes weight loss resistance. You will find quizzes to help you prioritize which systems to work on, and you will discover what to do to overcome your personal obstacles.

This book is not only theoretical though, because without *supported* action, you will never sustain changes in your body. You will also find tips and tricks, a 30-day step-by-step implementation plan, and three meal plan levels to meet you where you are. Everything you need to get the results you want!

What This Book Is Not

I want to get this out of the way before you can sneak another skeptical eye roll. This book is not directed at those who are a size 1 trying to get to a size 0. I am not here to tell you there is anything wrong with that, but you will not find your solutions between these covers. This book is not a magic bullet. It will not involve you starving yourself; you will not be white knuckling it through your day. This plan does not rely on you eating five to six meals per day. There are no obscure ingredients or recipes that you need a chef to prepare. You do not have to take pills to achieve your goals. You will not be dropping weight quickly and gaining it back even quicker. You will not be shamed into success. This is not a yo-yo diet.

It is so much more! The ultimate goal is for you to personalize your plan, to understand your body and to bust weight loss myths for good.

My Story

Weight loss resistance was my identity for decades. I was never a healthy kid: my poor mother dealt with infection after infection, skin rashes, pneumonia, and digestive and sleep troubles throughout my childhood. Alongside all these issues, I also faced persistent weight gain. It wasn't for lack of trying to lose weight either. My mother took me from appointment to appointment, seeing dieticians, getting lab work done, enrolling me in sports and other activities. It never quite made sense why I was obese. My medical doctor, doing the best he could, would always say, "Well if it's not broken, don't fix it." But I *felt* broken.

As I entered my early teens, my health concerns continued to escalate. At this point I had been diagnosed with juvenile rheumatoid arthritis, I had crippling digestive problems and ongoing surgeries for ear issues, injuries, etc. My weight continued to creep up no matter how little I ate, and at this point all of my doctors were pressuring me to lose weight. They would not believe that I was actually eating as little as I said or that I was as active as I told them. They said it was impossible to be the weight I was while doing "all the right things." I was accused of binging, overeating, sneaking food, and so forth. I remember these demoralizing discussions as if they happened yesterday.

There is a silver lining to this story though, or I wouldn't be writing this book. When I was about 16 years old, one of my co-workers went on Oprah's "no whites" diet. He started to see great results and shared his secret with me. Having tried probably a hundred different diets at this point, I was skeptical at best, but I felt so horrible that I decided to try it. This was my first experience with food as medicine and the first time that I realized the *type* of food I put in my body had a significant impact on my health. My digestive problems started to improve, along with my skin issues and joint pain. I even saw my weight slowly change. This gave me the confidence to believe in my body again, to start to move differently, and to view my lifestyle through a different lens. That was until an awful virus tore my system down, bringing me to the next leg of my journey (the final one to be discussed here—the rest is for another book).

After not recovering amidst months of illness and sleeping 23 hours a day, my mother took me to the naturopathic doctor in town as a last-ditch effort. We lived in a small town, and this was back when naturopathic medicine was perceived as fringe medicine! My ND began to teach me about how food interacts with the body, how our genetics affect us, and also about the sources and outcomes of inflammation. I was *captivated*! She also pushed me to have further blood work and investigations to help better understand my chronic fatigue, inflammation, and weight loss resistance. I was already hooked, but as she helped me further to have celiac disease diagnosed and to understand the importance of gut health and hormones, I knew this was the type of medicine that I had to practice.

Now a fully licensed ND, I see patients every day who are dealing with similar struggles. My role is to take all of their symptoms to put the puzzle pieces together, not only to explain the true underlying links among them but also to empower my patients to figure out the key activities that will help them to maintain lifelong health. I wrote this book as a way to help more women than I can feasibly reach in my office. My goal is to help women overcome all the misperceptions about weight loss.

Do You Have Weight Loss Resistance?

The number one sign of weight loss resistance is embarking on diet after diet with little to no results. Myself, I had tried the Mediterranean diet, a low-fat diet, Weight Watchers, a vegetarian diet, the vegetable soup diet, and many more.

Other physical signs of weight loss resistance include:
- stubborn weight loss around the abdomen,
- skin tag development or changes to skin pigmentation,
- digestive discomfort (bloating, gas, constipation, or diarrhea),
- difficulty falling or staying asleep,
- difficulty waking up or fatigue throughout the day,
- joint aches and pains,
- anxiety that cycles throughout the day,
- food cravings and intense feelings of being driven by food reward/ punishment,
- feelings of getting "hangry" (so hungry you feel angry) between meals and needing snacks to stabilize your focus, concentration, energy, and mood, and
- the sense that all you need is one more ounce of willpower to achieve your goals.

Other medical conditions important to the discussion of weight loss resistance include:
- type 2 diabetes,
- fatty liver disease,
- elevated cholesterol or triglycerides,
- sleep apnea,
- polycystic ovarian syndrome (PCOS), or
- gut infections.

Throughout this book, you'll find that I discuss real patient cases, although names and personal details have been changed to protect privacy. These are people who were previously struggling, just like you.

"I SWEAR, NO ONE BELIEVES ME, BUT I AM DOING EVERYTHING RIGHT. I AM NOT LYING, I AM NOT BINGING ON FOOD. WHAT IS WRONG WITH ME?"

Anna, a former model, prided herself on her appearance, her discipline, and her health. After Anna had children, she found that her old tricks to lose weight weren't working. She would creep up 5 lbs here, 10 lbs there, and after two children she was 50 lbs heavier than her former self. Anna worked out when she could, although her stressful job and busy home life prevented a consistent schedule. She was sacrificing her sleep to fit things in, and as a result she was getting recurring infections and taking multiple rounds of antibiotics. When I saw Anna, she was beside herself, restricting her calories to less than 1,000 per day. She had just adopted a vegetarian diet as a last desperate effort to meet her weight loss goals. She told me she was seconds away from weight loss surgery! Anna was a mess, her health was poor, but the first thing she said as she sat in my office was, "I swear, no one believes me, but I am doing everything right. I am not lying, I am not binging on food. What is wrong with me?"

Many of you will recognize pieces of your own story in Anna's. You are in the right place to change that story!

Setting the Record Straight

What you have been told about weight loss is *wrong*! But you already know that from your results, or rather lack of results. Naturally, everyone has opinions, but looking deep into the science is the goal of this book. There is none of the indecisiveness of, "Eggs are good. No wait, they are bad. Oops, we were wrong again; they are good." We will get into the facts. What we are facing is a hormone issue—a physiology issue. No amount of calories will get you out of that predicament, and restricting calories can even make the issues worse.

The Diet-Free Dials—A Sneak Peek

When you have something that is "undiagnosable," or just a general feeling of awful, there is very little that the conventional medical system can do for you. This is no fault of its own either. Much of the training revolves around the pathology model—a sickness model—approach to healthcare. In order to understand my own health issues I have had to dive into an understanding of the wellness model. What does it take to be well? What does it take to perform optimally, have a clear head, endless energy, smooth digestion, and a small waistline?

I've learned that wellness takes a deep understanding of what I call the diet-free dials. These dials need to be in just the right position to experience effortless weight loss and wellness. But that does not mean we need to work on adjusting all of them at the same time. Life-change stress is still stress, so we'll break down the changes into manageable pieces together.

Weight Loss Potential

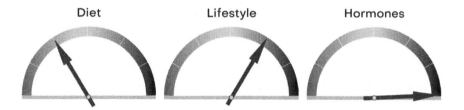

Figure 1. These dials represent all the factors that need to be working optimally for weight loss to occur. What you eat is an important part of weight loss, but considered alone it will not provide the benefits you hope for. To unlock your fat-burning potential, attention to lifestyle components, such as sleep and circadian rhythm, stress, and meal timing, and hormones also must come into play through various mechanisms.

Sleep and Circadian Rhythms

Falling under the rubric of the lifestyle dial, these are technically two separate dials, but sleep and the circadian rhythm truly need to be discussed together. We all know what sleep is (especially if we aren't getting enough of it), but what the heck is the circadian rhythm? Well, the circadian rhythm is your body's internal clock. It sends signals about when we should be awake, when we should be asleep, when our metabolic hormones should be resetting (aka when we burn fat), how well our immune system is controlled, and the list goes on.

(i) **Metabolic hormones** are substances—peptides or steroids—that are made in various endocrine tissues, such as your pancreas, digestive tract, adrenal gland, brain, and many other tissues. These travel in the bloodstream and affect your metabolic rate and which fuel you burn (protein, fat, or sugar). Examples include leptin, insulin, GLP, and cortisol.

An increasing number of researchers are investigating the effects of the circadian rhythm on hormonal balance, weight loss, and inflammatory levels. We will explore these relationships and more aspects relating to how to work *with* your circadian rhythm, and look at all the ways you are currently working *against* it!

You not only need adequate sleep, but you also need to sleep at the right time, which is dictated by circadian rhythm, for your metabolic hormones to signal properly and to see the benefits of losing weight effortlessly. Eating in alignment with your circadian rhythm is also a significant piece to understand: if you eat the right food at the wrong time of day it will actually cause you to gain fat.

Adjusting the dials for sleep and circadian rhythm changes can provide the greatest impact when it comes to changing weight loss resistance. If you are not working on it, then it is working against you—and you are losing the struggle!

Stress

Before you roll your eyes with a "here we go again" attitude, we need to recognize that stress is about so much more than the tension you feel and your perception of life events. The stress that your body has to deal with also includes hidden stressors, such as blood sugar swings, hormonal imbalance, underlying infections, inflammation, disease, food intolerances, sleep disturbance, and many other factors unique to you. We need to take a whole body approach to treating the stressors in our lives. I know first-hand that weight both piles on and sticks like a magnet in stressful situations.

Here's a bird's-eye view into why. In the face of a stressor, cortisol is released from the adrenal gland along with norepinephrine and epinephrine (aka adrenaline). Cortisol can act to increase blood sugar levels (so that you have energy to run from a bear, for example). This increase in blood sugar also primes your metabolic hormones, specifically insulin, to leap into action. The elevation in insulin helps to shuttle the blood sugar out of the blood and into the fat cells to protect us from high blood sugar. Here's the kicker: this stress response also happens when you are sitting at your desk all day long—without a bear in sight. Meaning? You are stuck in fat storage mode! Cortisol also controls your inflammation levels, your neurotransmitters, your hormonal balance and your digestion. It's a powerful hormone.

Insulin is a metabolic hormone that protects the body from high blood sugar. When blood sugar increases with a meal, insulin comes in and binds the receptor, lowering blood sugar and storing it away as glycogen in your muscles, liver, and fat cells. This makes energy available during periods of starvation. (As you read this book, you'll come to see that our bodies are hard-wired for self-preservation.) Insulin is a key hormone to understand because issues with insulin signalling have a lot to do with weight loss resistance.

We will delve into all of these aspects about stress response and insulin function throughout the discussion in **chapter 4 and 6**, as well as covering actionable strategies, supplements, and small changes to help deal with stress and prevent its detrimental effects—even when stress is inevitable.

"AS MUCH AS 60% OF YOUR INSULIN RELEASE IS DETERMINED IN YOUR GUT! YOU KNOW WHAT THAT MEANS, HOW QUICKLY YOU STORE FAT AND HOW EASY IT IS TO LOSE STARTS RIGHT HERE."

Gut Bacteria and Hormones

The bacteria in your gut also have critical roles to play in weight loss. Gut bacteria determine your cravings, how much energy you extract from the food you eat, how well you detox your hormones, and even how well your metabolic hormones are regulated. As much as 60% of your insulin release is determined in your gut! You know what that means, how quickly you store fat and how easy it is to lose it starts right here. We have all felt the effects of inflammation in the body, aches and pains, anxiety and depression, bloating, and water weight. These are all regulated by our digestive system.

Many a wise doctor has said that health starts in the gut. I agree with that! If you are not digesting, absorbing, and eliminating properly, you will feel crappy (I couldn't resist the pun!)—and your weight will reflect that.

Metabolic Hormones

To tie it all together, we will explore how all the above factors affect our master fat-regulating hormones, which include insulin, leptin, growth hormone, hunger hormones, and fullness hormones. What you need to know here is that the dance between these hormones can completely make or break your experience with food and weight regulation. From my clinical experience, most people are controlled by their metabolic hormones, not the other way around!

Do you get "hangry" (so hungry that you feel angry) throughout the day? Do you *need* snacks and get shaky and overwhelmed when you don't eat? Does sugar give you a pick-me-up? Do you feel sleepy after eating? If so, my friend, you rely on sugar to keep you going, and you also likely have a limited capacity to use your fat as fuel. For those who want to scream, "Use my fat! I have pounds and pounds of it available," what you don't know is that the padlocks are on your fat cells. Yes, the issue is that your body is using sugar, or carbohydrates, to keep your blood sugar stable. You are not in fat-burning mode. This cycle must be reversed in order to achieve your weight loss goals, regulate your appetite, and use all of those body fat stores to fuel your day!

"MOST PEOPLE ARE CONTROLLED BY THEIR METABOLIC HORMONES, NOT THE OTHER WAY AROUND!"

Mindset

When you have struggled with weight loss resistance, just thinking about weight loss again can be difficult. Many women express to me that they feel like a failure, they don't have the willpower to start, and they don't trust their bodies. The reality is many of you have never been taught how to think for success, how to program your minds, establish consistent habits, and figure out which lifestyle change will provide you with the long-term results you desire. This critical piece pertaining to mindset is missing from most programs, but not here!

Take Action
Small win changes are essential. This book has a lot to say about habit formation tactics and how to achieve your goals. The key to any of that is taking action, which is exactly what I want you to get used to doing as

we move through this book. So why not get started! Before diving in, it's important to consider the time you are going to dedicate to food and lifestyle changes and the support systems you have in place.

The reality is, if I'm learning a new sport or a new language, it takes time. It doesn't take a lot of time, but at least 30 minutes of my day is dedicated to that task. Now, look at your calendar for the upcoming week and see if there are three to four 15–30-minute blocks where you can read this book. Put those reminders in your calendar to hold yourself accountable.

In **chapter 1** we will also be covering the importance of accountability and partners with you on this journey. For now, start thinking of who those people might be and brainstorm your list.

THIS BOOK WILL ACT AS YOUR ROAD MAP, OUTLINING WHAT YOU NEED TO KNOW TO UNDERSTAND WHAT YOUR BODY IS TELLING YOU, WHY YOU ARE HOLDING ON TO WEIGHT YOU DON'T WANT OR NEED, AND HOW TO BEGIN TO BREAK THE CYCLE OF WEIGHT LOSS RESISTANCE.

The Rules of Engagement

I recognize that the dials discussed above have likely excited you, because there is now hope that something fixable may be going on with you! That said, I have put enough women through this program to know that you are also asking, "Before I say yes to this, what is this plan actually going to look like?" For this reason, I have developed the Rules of Engagement, the Yes/No list that this program is based around. Throughout the course of this book, we will be diving deep into the *why* behind each of these items and uncovering just how you need to personalize your program for success.

The *Finally* Lose It Program

Say yes to:

Stocking whole foods. Delicious, simple, easy to find whole foods.

Thinking about when and how you eat. As much as diet, i.e., the foods you choose, is a cornerstone of this plan, when and how you eat are also critical factors in overcoming your weight loss resistance. This book will teach you how to personalize timing and approach to meals in the Finally Lose It Program.

Personalizing your plan. Everything in this program needs to be customized to you. That is why you'll find quizzes throughout the book and a laboratory blood work guide at the back so that you can work with a medical practitioner to get to the bottom of your health concerns.

Getting adequate sleep and reducing stress. Frankly, you will need to be taught how important quality sleep and stress reduction are if you want to meet your goals and sustain your progress. Many women are never taught how to reduce their stress or support their sleep; these are foundational pieces to the Finally Lose It Program.

Checking your mindset. Adopt a growth mindset. Accept new challenges. Look at how you have gone about weight loss in the past, and change your views and your habits. These elements are not often discussed in weight loss books, but they have proven to be pivotal to the ongoing success of every woman who has been through the Finally Lose It Program.

Say no to:

A "no pain, no gain" mentality. This program is not hard. I promise you have been through much harder things in life, even much harder programs. When you are stressed to the nines and then you add the stress of another fad diet, it's no wonder that you don't see the results you have hoped for. Weight loss doesn't have to be painful.

Making excuses. Excuses, simply put, are broken promises to yourself. They offer nothing except a feeling of failure and incompetence. Over time, you have likely learned to take them on as opportunities for your mindset gremlins to step in and prove to you that you can't do it, you aren't good enough, and that you shouldn't try again. Lose these excuses on Day 1. In Finally Lose It you will learn how to work with your habit forming type. You will not feel suffocated by this health plan and we offer accountability to boot.

Eating cardboard "diet" food. You never have to eat tasteless, funky ingredient-filled, gross food anymore. I mean it! Don't eat food that you do not like. Don't like Brussels sprouts? Don't eat them! When food becomes a forced experience, you will never sustain the results, and you will crave more junk foods.

Eating inflammatory and addictive foods. Sugar, artificial sweeteners, industrial seed oils, food additives, alcohol, wheat, dairy, and grains will be cut out for 30 days in phase 3. These foods interact with your brain to aggravate cravings, and they also can cause inflammation in your brain, gut, and metabolic system. Both of these factors, cravings and inflammation, exacerbate weight loss resistance.

Complicated shopping lists, meal plans, and overwhelming meal prep. There are few things that frustrate me more than a shopping list four pages long, spending hours in the grocery store looking for obscure ingredients, and spending hundreds of dollars at the cash register, only to get home to use 1 tsp. of an ingredient, and then the rest ends up going bad. I have developed a system for meal preparation that focuses on delicious ingredients, simple preparation, and a shopping list that fits on a Post-it note!

Finally Lose It Program Design

As someone who has been where you are now, I am determined to help get women talking and sharing about weight loss struggles in a community. You would be shocked by who else in your life is also silently suffering in isolation. My goal with this book it to bring women together to learn about their bodies, develop book clubs and online and in-person support groups to build each other up.

Combining naturopathic medicine with a job in obesity research allows me to bring you this streamlined, no-nonsense, evidence-based approach to understand your health and weight loss resistance as a side effect of an unhealthy body. This book will act as your road map, outlining what you need to know to understand what your body is telling you, why you are holding on to weight you don't want or need, and how to begin to break the cycle of weight loss resistance. I truly want nothing more than for you to achieve your health goals and to join the countless women who have regained their health—body, mind, and spirit—through a greater understanding of the right hormonal balance, the right foods at the right times, with the right support (lifestyle, habits, supplements, etc.).

This won't be *easy*, but it will be much easier than the stuff you've been putting yourself through up to this point. It is also a lot easier than facing a life with type 2 diabetes, crippling fatigue, premature aging, sleep apnea/disturbance, arthritis, other autoimmune diseases, and debilitating and embarrassing digestive issues. And it is easier than living a life driven by cravings, low self-esteem, and all of the self-imposed missed opportunities.

Let's end this "one diet, one plan, one nutrient to solve everyone's problems" mentality. There are 7 billion diets for 7 billion people. It is my intention to help you, as a busy professional woman, to regain trust and faith in your body and embrace your health potential like I have, with a completely different outlook, fewer joint pains and digestive issues, a strong immune system, energy to spare, and 80 lbs (you fill in your own number!) lighter. Your life is waiting! You truly cannot afford to *not* go through this system. Turn the page, and let's get started.

A love note about the terms pounds lost and diet
You will occasionally read about X person losing X pounds in this book. (It is a weight loss book after all.) But you need to know that how you feel in your body is more important than a number on a scale. In fact, I do not encourage weighing yourself. Truthfully, many of my patients see success but have no idea what the "number" was because their body image issues would flare up if they so much as stepped beside a scale.

I'm sure you've had the experience of feeling super lean and sexy one day, you really feel like you're rocking it, and then you step on the scale to see that nothing has changed. This can ruin your whole day and throw you into a self-hating "what I eat doesn't matter anyway" spiral. No one deserves that, and it will not happen on my watch. Measure your waist and hips if you want, watch the pant sizes drop and your shirts start to hang off you, but don't judge your success based on an arbitrary number, unless you truly have no emotional attachment to it. (Because, let's be honest ladies, anything that can change 5–10 lbs based on where you are in your menstrual cycle just can't be trusted!)

Diet, which literally means "style of eating," likely has a lot of negative connotations for you. Understandably so. I get it. You have tried just about every style of eating and still haven't achieved your goals. You will see the word diet used throughout this book. As much as this is a style of eating that I will be asking you to follow, it is also much more than that. This approach is not a short-term restriction or abuse pattern to help you lose weight, only to gain it back again. The Finally Lose It Program is about less restriction, more nourishment, and correcting your physiology. It is about a choice to be healthier and to give up the fight against your body.

PART ONE

The Finally Lose It Education Plan
Metabolism 101

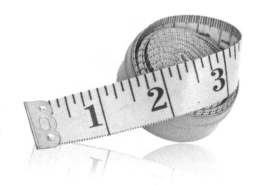

YESTERDAY YOU SAID TOMORROW.

—UNKNOWN (AKA **ALL OF US!**)

1

WHY DIETS FAIL

Now that you have started the book, I bet you are feeling hopeful, feeling as if you may be heard for the first time, or that success might actually be possible for you. I am here to assure you that it is! We have to set some ground rules though, so that you don't fall into the same traps as you have in the past. I believe that awareness comes in breakthroughs, so before we set you up for success, let's address the problems with typical diets that set you up for failure. I want you to reread this chapter any time you feel like you are slipping or falling off of the proverbial wagon. When you can identify the obstacle you are facing, you can easily identify the coping strategy to overcome it.

Problem: The other diet was too strict.

Solution: If you are struggling through it, feeling deprived, and socially isolating yourself so that you can try to lose weight, then you are bound to give in to temptation. The reality is, eating a meal out of your house once per week likely won't completely throw off all of your success on this plan. In fact, it can be much more psychologically supportive to *plan* a meal out. This sort of variety may actually support your physiology as well, keeping your body from becoming complacent and hitting a plateau. In this book, we will explore the importance of loosening the belt and not holding on for dear life to your diet plan. A rigid plan can also lead to an all-or-nothing mindset, which is challenging—and discouraging—to sustain.

Problem: You have an all-or-nothing mindset.

Solution: How many times on a diet have you given in to the chocolate cake, french fries, or potato chips, and then said, "Screw it! If I ate that, then I might as well eat everything else I want!" This is a classic example of the all-or-nothing (on the diet or off of the diet) mindset that will keep you in trouble. It also sends you into a shame spiral; you start hating on yourself, and you lose more and more confidence in your body's ability to succeed. This is one of the hardest mindset shifts to make because the response is so deeply ingrained by our society. Defending yourself from thinking perfectionism is the way to go will be critical. And when you understand your body and know what you can get away with, you will feel so much more confident in making decisions that are good for your mind *and* your waistline! No more black and white because we all prefer the shades of grey, don't we?

"IT IS NOT ONLY HOW MUCH YOU EAT THAT DETERMINES YOUR WEIGHT LOSS BUT ALSO HOW THAT FOOD AFFECTS THE HORMONAL BALANCE OF YOUR BODY."

Problem: You focused on calories.

Solution: If you thought calories were the be-all and end-all with regard to weight loss, and if it worked for you, you would not be here. The concept that calories in must equal calories out is the biggest urban myth out there. It is a disgrace to our bodies as well. As if we were that naïve! Consider how people survive famines. Your body can adjust the amount of calories it burns to keep it proportional to the calories consumed. This is why you become exhausted, cold, and hungry when you are on a diet. Everything in your body slows down to protect you. And how does it slow down? Hormones are the culprit here. That is why it is not only how much you eat that determines your weight loss but also how that food affects the hormonal balance of your body. We will explore this relationship further on.

Problem: You rely on willpower.

Solution: There is truly nothing quite like starving and battling your way through the day. Willpower is a finite resource to the body. We wake up with a full tank, but going through the day facing temptation after temptation, resisting our hunger urges, and planning what to eat next and when depletes that tank. This is why the sugar monster feels at its most aggressive late in the evening, and why overeating even good food is likely to happen when you are tired and parked in front of the TV. With this book, not only will we focus on planning meals and setting rules for yourself that take the questioning out of the matter, but I will also show you the willpower-building activities that can keep you feeling craving- and deprivation-free throughout the day. No cardboard food here! You will be nourished *and* eat delicious food.

Problem: You don't know your *true* motivation.

Solution: Here's the reality of the matter: if you only want to lose weight to fit into a bathing suit, it is going to be harder for you to follow this plan and keep the weight off. We need to have a deeply motivating why. For me, I wanted to get my energy and physical performance capacity back. I wanted to figure things out so that I could share my discoveries with the world to try to help prevent anyone from feeling how I had felt in my body.

For many of my patients, their *why* is so that they can play with their kids more, ask for a promotion, have more endurance, or feel really sexy naked! Even those are somewhat superficial examples, compared to when you dive deep into why you *truly* want to lose weight. And that is what you need to have plastered up on your wall, because that is what will make tough choices become easy. If I am having a ton of cravings and really just want that second, or third, piece of dark chocolate, it is very easy to ask myself if that fits with my mission to change the world, woman by woman. The answer is obviously no, and I move on to walking, reading, or stretching until the craving passes.

Problem: You have unhealthy expectations.

Solution: I mentioned in the beginning that if you are looking to go from a size 1 to a size 0 then this book is not for you. Well, the same is true if you are looking to go from a size 20 to a size 0 in six months. On another note, if you are 6 ft. tall and think your ideal weight is 100 lbs, think again. That is just not going to happen either, especially if you have a goal of becoming more fit. There is just no healthy way to achieve either of these extreme goals, and if that is what you are hoping for, no diet will provide that for you. Any diet is likely to fail with such unreasonable expectations. You will lose weight here, but it will be steady and consistent. You will feel better in your body and sustain it, but it will not happen overnight. The process does take patience.

WHEN I RAN LONG DISTANCE IN THE PAST, DO YOU THINK I JUST GOT UP AND RAN A HALF MARATHON? No WAY! AND IT WOULD SOUND ABSURD IF I TOLD YOU THAT WAS MY PLAN, NOW WOULDN'T IT? YET SOMEHOW THIS IS WHAT WE DO TO OURSELVES OVER AND OVER AGAIN!

Problem: If you fail to plan, you plan to fail.

This. Is. So. Critical. When I ran long distance in the past, do you think I just got up and ran a half marathon? No way! And it would sound absurd if I told you that was my plan, now wouldn't it? Yet somehow this is what we do to ourselves over and over again! Once you fix on the idea that you want to lose weight, you probably even choose a type of diet you are going to follow. Let's say, for example, it is a low-carb diet. You will look up what carbs are, convince yourself it won't be too bad eliminating those foods, and maybe you even get a meal plan to support you. This may sound like a complete plan, but this is why I see patients fail so often.

When setting a weight loss plan, and to set yourself up for success, the other questions you must be asking yourself include: what events do I have coming up that I need to plan for? What items do I need to get out of my house? What are my staple meals going to be when I am too busy to cook? What can I eat when I forget my lunch? When are my mealtimes going to be? What am I going to feed my family?

What days will I meal prep? When will I make time to sleep? How will I deal with stress? Will I work out? The list goes on and on, and we'll get into that later on, but these examples clarify what I mean by "planning."

If you do not have someone supporting you with a plan, or if you only think about what food items you need to eat, then you have missed 80% of what you need to actually succeed! This is one of my main critiques of most health books: they leave you with all this amazing information, but then you have no idea how to act on it, or where to start. The thirty-day start-up guide in **chapter 9** is my attempt to ensure that doesn't happen for you.

Problem: You don't have enough support.

Solution: There is a reason that so many of us flock to group programs and social media groups. We need community! Feeling part of a community is not only about the mindset of feeling like you are a part of something and that other people are going through the same struggles as you, but there is also a neurological response at work. When you see someone else succeed, you see how they do it and you're on the path with them, then what happens in your brain is incredible. We have neurons, or brain cells, called *mirror neurons* that sense not only your actions and intentions but also those of the people around you. It is called *group as a whole* mentality. This is automatically programmed, so to be honest it either works with you, or against you. If you have friends or family members who do not support you, it will be a much harder road to make lifestyle changes.

Picture yourself in a group of like-minded women, all working toward the same goal. You're mirror neurons are working with you here because the group is moving forward and succeeding together. This is so essential that I have a whole package for you to share with friends or family members who you want to bring on board with you. If you go to **www.sarahwilsonnd.com/loseitbookbonus** you will see the Accountability Partner package. In here I have a script on how to ask for support, a video walking your chosen support partners through the program basics, and sample chapters for them to read. It is critical to have a group, so don't miss out on these bonuses.

If you want to achieve your goals, lose the weight, and have the journey feel less lonely and overwhelming, then lend your book to someone when you are done, gift them a copy, or download the free program overview and share it in your group. Community is a game changer.

Problem: You do not have enough accountability.

Solution: Support and accountability can go hand in hand when they work well. An accountability partner's job is to help you set goals and then firmly hold you to them. This candidate is loving and supportive, but this person will also call you on your excuses and be a neutral sounding board. This is why I often recommend choosing a large support network and only one accountability partner, which may even be outside of that network. You do not want to choose your best friend who always tells you that you are perfect, no matter what. That person is critical to bring on board as a support team member, but she is not the person you should report to when you have eaten a whole pan of brownies because you got in a fight with your partner. In those cases, you need tough love. For many people, their accountability partner is a naturopathic doctor, nutritionist, or personal trainer. Skipping this step often leads to falling off after you hit the first obstacle. That is the last thing I want for you.

"IF YOU HAVE A BIG OL' BRICK ON YOUR METABOLISM THAT IS BLOCKING YOUR WEIGHT LOSS SUCCESS, THEN OF COURSE EVERYDAY STRATEGIES WILL FAIL."

Take Action

Before going any further, refer to the list you've made of people you want in your support group and consider who might be a good accountability partner for you. I want you to send that person an email with the information from the Accountability Partner package from **www.sarahwilsonnd.com/loseitbookbonus**.

Problem: There are underlying obstacles.

Solution: If you have a big ol' brick on your metabolism that is blocking your weight loss success, then of course everyday strategies will fail. The most common underlying obstacles include gut issues, inflammation, circadian rhythm and sleep concerns, stress, insulin resistance, toxicity, and thyroid issues. These are covered in the book. (For still more in-depth information on thyroid health and toxicity, check out my website at sarahwilsonnd.com for the latest blog posts.)

Are you feeling ready for the next steps? I hope you are excited! Now that you know the biggest pitfalls to avoid on your journey to health, it's time to dive into the nitty-gritty of getting you well. In the next chapter, I discuss the first piece of the puzzle, the circadian rhythm. If you're not in tune with your body's natural rhythms, you're missing out on a powerful weight loss mechanism.

SMALL SHIFTS
IN YOUR THINKING, AND
SMALL CHANGES IN YOUR
ENERGY, CAN LEAD TO
MASSIVE ALTERATIONS
OF YOUR END RESULT.

—KEVIN MICHEL

2

FIND YOUR RHYTHM

The circadian rhythm is your body's internal 24-hour clock. When it is working well, it knows when you should be awake, when you should be asleep, when to burn fat, and when to store fat. Working with your body's internal rhythm is one of the most foundational concepts of the Finally Lose It Program. If your body doesn't know when to sleep, when to make digestive juices, when to clean up your immune system, and when to reset your metabolism, then your body becomes a construction crew without a foreman. It is in a state of chaos, and your goals to build a healthier body just go down the tubes.

"But I am a night owl, Dr. Sarah! I think the best and get my best work done after 10:00 p.m."

Kennedy worked as a pediatric nurse, a job that she loved. She loved caring for children when they came in, comforting them and their parents through the difficult illnesses they would be facing. When Kennedy came into my office, the first thing she said to me was that something felt "off." She knew she was overweight, but no matter how hard she tried, she couldn't seem to lose those extra pounds, and every year more would pile on. She was exhausted and spending her spare time using her own medical knowledge to research what could be happening to her. Doctor Google told her it might be her thyroid or it might be her hormones. She thought her metabolism was slow, so she started to work out on her lunch breaks and eat five to six small meals per day. Kennedy came into my office, begging me to provide her with a list of testing that might help to get to the root of what was happening.

What I found out next changed the course of my eventual treatment. Although Kennedy took great pride in a job she loved to her core and did not find it stressful in any way, it became clear over the course of our visit that in order to serve her pediatric patients, her job involved shift work.

Kennedy began her nursing career at the age of 25. She had always been proud of herself throughout university, as she worked hard to eat relatively healthy and keep the "freshman 15" at bay. She always had to work to maintain her weight, but she saw the results of her efforts. Within months of starting shift work, Kennedy found that she felt "puffy." Maybe she was just retaining water, she thought, or maybe it was the change in food at her job. Her boyfriend at the time said he did not notice any changes, so she thought it might be in her head and carried on. One year in, she could not button up her jeans, and she knew something was up! She decided to go on a diet with her sister. The diet turned out to be a mostly vegetarian juicing diet. Keeping full on juice, potatoes, sweet potatoes, bananas, and other fruits, Kennedy found that she actually gained weight on this diet! How was that even possible when her sister was losing a few pounds a week?

Subsequently, Kennedy tried diet after diet. Nothing seemed to work for her; she was exasperated. Fast forward four years and Kennedy was in my office, preparing for her wedding and desperate to figure out what could be wrong. When we began to talk about her meals in the run of a week, I discovered they alternated: four days she would eat five to six meals throughout the night at work, and the other three days she ate her meals with her fiancé. Kennedy's "lunchtime" workouts were actually occurring at midnight in the gym beside the hospital. She loved these workouts because the gym was quiet and it woke her up halfway through the night. What Kennedy did not love was what I had to tell her. Her issue may not be related to her thyroid or even that she needed to work out more and eat less. What Kennedy needed to learn more about was how her circadian rhythm, or 24-hour clock, was affecting her metabolism.

"IF YOU WERE ON THE PERFECT CIRCADIAN CYCLE (WHICH FEW PEOPLE ARE IN THE WESTERN WORLD), THEN YOU WOULD BE HUNGRY ONLY WHEN YOUR BODY NEEDED FOOD AND WITHOUT CRAVINGS; YOU WOULD HAVE LOW ENVIRONMENTAL STRESS LEVELS; YOU WOULD SLEEP SOUNDLY AND WAKE REFRESHED; YOU WOULD HAVE LOW LEVELS OF INFLAMMATION AND RESIST PREMATURE AGING; AND YOU WOULD HAVE HARMONIOUS FAT BURNING."

What Is the Circadian Rhythm?

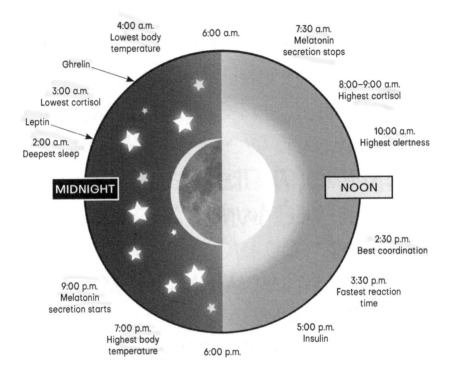

Figure 2. Our body's natural rhythms are controlled by the daily variations of light and dark. This is our sleep-wake cycle, which (for most) is related to the cycle of the sun. The release of melatonin around 9:00 p.m. makes us feel sleepy in the evening, and its cessation in the early hours of the morning coincides with cortisol increases which help us wake up as the day begins. Sleep-wake and other daily patterns seen here are part of our circadian rhythms, (*circum* means "around" and *dies* "day"). These cycles, governed by the body's internal or biological clock housed deep within the brain, adaptively organize the body's daily functions into near 24-hour oscillations termed *circadian rhythms*.

The circadian rhythm is the twenty-four-hour clock in the body that determines many of our biological functions, such as when we wake up, when we fall asleep, when our digestion is primed, when we move the most, when our immune system is active; it can even control our metabolism and other hormones. The circadian rhythm is influenced by many different signals, the main ones being light and dark cycles, food intake, and periods of movement and exercise.

Light is a particularly strong signal. After it enters our eyes, it interacts with an area of our brain known as the suprachiasmatic nucleus (SCN), where light signals the SCN that it's daytime. The body then anticipates how awake you need to be, when you digest, what temperature will be just right, and essentially controls all the differences between our awake and our asleep body. Research in this area is constantly evolving, but we know that eating, hormone release, inflammation control, and even fat burning versus fat storage can be determined by this force.[1]

The Suprachiasmatic Nucleus
Controls Your Hormones

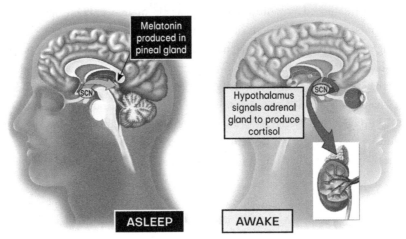

Melatonin produced in pineal gland

SCN

Hypothalamus signals adrenal gland to produce cortisol

SCN

ASLEEP

AWAKE

SCN = Suprachiasmatic nucleus

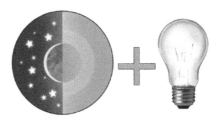

Figure 3. The cycles of the circadian rhythm are coordinated by the suprachiasmatic nucleus. This part of your brain synchronizes your hormones to the changing cycles of light and dark. Things like jet lag, shift work, and excess screen time late at night can throw this cycle off-kilter. When this happens, your physical and mental health can suffer.

If you were on the perfect circadian cycle (which few people are in the Western world), you would be hungry only when your body needed food and without cravings; you would have low environmental stress levels; you would sleep soundly and wake refreshed; you would have low levels of inflammation and resist premature aging; and you would have harmonious fat burning. Obviously, our circadian rhythm does not exist in isolation, and there is overlap between this and other systems (hence this book). What we do know is that even in isolation, altered circadian rhythms can have a profound impact.

How is it possible that Kennedy, for instance, started to gain weight out of nowhere? Well, research shows that those who are subjected to shift work have an increased body mass, increased blood glucose levels, increased plasma lipids, and increased triglycerides, which can be markers of insulin resistance.[1] All of this is independent of the total amount of food consumed. These results are not unique to a specific population of night-shift workers either. It doesn't matter if you are a nurse, a security guard, or a factory worker. It doesn't matter if you are stressed at work, love working shifts, or hate working shifts. All of the studies show a similar outcome.

On a personal note, my research into shift work–induced circadian issues did not come from my own experience but was triggered by a drive to understand the root causes of my father's health concerns, and also the patterns that I saw in the parents of my friends. Being from a small town, many people worked in factories and 24-hour industries. I witnessed the frustration and health demise of so many people for "no good reason." The years of shift work were taking a toll, and something didn't feel quite right to me.

As I began to see patients, both in that small town and now in a big city that never sleeps, I saw patient after patient who had long-standing issues with their metabolism, digestion, immune system, and insomnia. So many of these people were just like Kennedy, or worse. They had metabolic syndrome (which consists of hypertension, insulin resistance, and obesity) long after they had finished their years of shift work. I believe that we are just now learning the true long-term effects that some of these careers have on the body. And we are learning how to correct some of them as well. The troubling part is that so many women have no idea that circadian dysregulation is the reason they are struggling with weight loss in the first place. With research and education, and groups of women coming together, women like Kennedy, night-shift workers who have become programmed to be at an increased risk of weight loss resistance, can stop beating themselves up about what they are eating and begin to understand their health in a bigger picture.

If you are thinking, I don't work shift work, so this doesn't apply to me, then think again! Circadian rhythm issues show up in many more subtle ways than just as a result of shift work. This is the area that I find totally and completely fascinating. I have always been a morning person. I have never had issues with sleeping until noon, unless I was very sick. I would often bounce out of bed, ready to start my day. As I am always on a self-improvement kick, I have tried many a productivity or health hack that involved timing of activities throughout the day: should I work out in the morning or at night, do my creative work in the morning or at night, eat early in the morning or fast until lunch? All of these strategies had an impact on my health, for better or for worse. As I started to trace out some of these patterns, everything clicked for me.

I was never able to lose weight on diets that emphasized snacks before bed. As recently as two years ago, I was exploring a bodybuilding-style diet that I can now see altered my circadian rhythm, altered my insulin production (which we will explore later), and led to the development of a strong but fluffier body. Even when I was running a half marathon, I would need to "fuel" myself the night before, and I gained weight during the process. The lesson here: you cannot outrun your circadian rhythms!

Assess Your Circadian Rhythm

As research is exploding in this area, we have more and more tools to accurately assess our own circadian rhythms. One of the mostly widely used is the "Morningness-Eveningness Questionnaire," which will give you a score that relates to your circadian rhythm type, also known as chronotype.[2]

1. Approximately what time would you get up if you were entirely free to plan your day?
[5] 5:00 a.m.–6:30 a.m. *(05:00–06:30 h)*
[4] 6:30 a.m.–7:45 a.m. *(06:30–07:45 h)*
[3] 7:45 a.m.–9:45 a.m. *(07:45–09:45 h)*
[2] 9:45 a.m.–11:00 a.m. *(09:45–11:00 h)*
[1] 11:00 a.m.–noon *(11:00–12:00 h)*

2. Approximately what time would you go to bed if you were entirely free to plan your evening?
[5] 8:00 p.m.–9:00 p.m. *(20:00–21:00 h)*
[4] 9:00 p.m.–10:15 p.m. *(21:00–22:15 h)*
[3] 10:15 p.m.–12:30 a.m. *(22:15–00:30 h)*
[2] 12:30 a.m.–1:45 a.m. *(00:30–01:45 h)*
[1] 1:45 a.m.–3:00 a.m. *(01:45–03:00 h)*

3. If you usually have to get up at a specific time in the morning, how much do you depend on an alarm clock?
[4] Not at all
[3] Slightly
[2] Somewhat
[1] Very much

4. How easy do you find it to get up in the morning (when you are not awakened unexpectedly)?

[1] Very difficult

[2] Somewhat difficult

[3] Fairly easy

[4] Very easy

5. How alert do you feel during the first half hour after you wake up in the morning?

[1] Not at all alert

[2] Slightly alert

[3] Fairly alert

[4] Very alert

6. How hungry do you feel during the first half hour after you wake up?

[1] Not at all hungry

[2] Slightly hungry

[3] Fairly hungry

[4] Very hungry

7. During the first half hour after you wake up in the morning, how do you feel?

[1] Very tired

[2] Fairly tired

[3] Fairly refreshed

[4] Very refreshed

8. If you had no commitments the next day, what time would you go to bed compared to your usual bedtime?

[4] Seldom or never later

[3] Less than 1 hour later

[2] 1–2 hours later

[1] More than 2 hours later

9. You have decided to do physical exercise. A friend suggests that you do this for one hour twice a week, and the best time for him is between 7:00 and 8:00 a.m. (07 and 08 h). Bearing in mind nothing but your own internal "clock," how do you think you would perform?

[4] Would be in good form

[3] Would be in reasonable form

[2] Would find it difficult

[1] Would find it very difficult

10. At approximately what time in the evening do you feel tired, and, as a result, in need of sleep?

[5] 8:00 p.m.–9:00 p.m. *(20:00–21:00 h)*

[4] 9:00 p.m.–10:15 p.m. *(21:00–22:15 h)*

[3] 10:15 p.m.–12:45 a.m. *(22:15–00:45 h)*

[2] 12:45 a.m.–2:00 a.m. *(00:45–02:00 h)*

[1] 2:00 a.m.–3:00 a.m. *(02:00–03:00 h)*

11. You want to be at your peak performance for a test that you know is going to be mentally exhausting and will last two hours. You are entirely free to plan your day. Considering only your internal "clock," which one of the four testing times would you choose?

[6] 8:00 a.m.–10:00 a.m. *(08:00–10:00 h)*

[4] 11:00 a.m.–1:00 p.m. *(11:00–13:00 h)*

[2] 3:00 p.m.–5:00 p.m. *(15:00–17:00 h)*

[0] 7:00 p.m.–9:00 p.m. *(19:00–21:00 h)*

12. If you got into bed at 11:00 PM (23:00 h), how tired would you be?

[0] Not at all tired

[2] A little tired

[3] Fairly tired

[5] Very tired

13. For some reason you have gone to bed several hours later than usual, but there is no need to get up at any particular time the next morning, which one of the following are you most likely to do?

[4] Will wake up at usual time, but will not fall back asleep

[3] Will wake up at usual time and will doze thereafter

[2] Will wake up at usual time, but will fall asleep again

[1] Will not wake up until later than usual

14. One night you have to remain awake between 4:00 and 6:00 a.m. (04:00 and 06:00 h) in order to carry out a night watch. You have no time commitments the next day. Which one of the alternatives would suit you best?

[1] Would not go to bed until the watch is over
[2] Would take a nap before and sleep after
[3] Would take a good sleep before and nap after
[4] Would sleep only before the watch

15. You have two hours of hard physical work. You are entirely free to plan your day. Considering only your internal "clock," which of the following times would you choose?

[4] 8:00 a.m.–10:00 a.m. *(08:00–10:00 h)*
[3] 11:00 a.m.–1:00 p.m. *(11:00–13:00 h)*
[2] 3:00 p.m.–5:00 p.m. *(15:00–17:00 h)*
[1] 7:00 p.m.–9:00 p.m. *(19:00–21:00 h)*

16. You have decided to do physical exercise. A friend suggests that you do this for one hour twice a week. The best time for her is between 10:00 and 11:00 p.m. (22:00 and23:00 h). Bearing in mind only your internal "clock," how well do you think you would perform?

[1] Would be in good form
[2] Would be in reasonable form
[3] Would find it difficult
[4] Would find it very difficult

17. Suppose you can choose your own work hours. Assume that you work a five-hour day (including breaks), your job is interesting, and you are paid based on your performance. At approximately what time would you choose to begin?

[5] 5 hours starting between 4:00 and 8:00 a.m. *(04:00–08:00 h)*
[4] 5 hours starting between 8:00 and 9:00 a.m. *(08:00–09:00 h)*
[3] 5 hours starting between 9:00 a.m. and 2:00 p.m. *(09:00–14:00 h)*
[2] 5 hours starting between 2:00 and 5:00 p.m. *(14:00–17:00 h)*
[1] 5 hours starting between 5:00 p.m.–4:00 a.m. *(17:00–04:00 h)*

18. At approximately what time of day do you usually feel your best?

[5] 5:00–8:00 a.m. *(05:00–08:00 h)*

[4] 8:00–10:00 a.m. *(08:00–10:00 h)*

[3] 10:00 a.m.–5:00 p.m. *(10:00–17:00 h)*

[2] 5:00–10:00 p.m. *(17:00–22:00 h)*

[1] 10:00 p.m.–5:00 a.m. *(22:00–05:00 h)*

19. One hears about "morning types" and "evening types." Which one of these types do you consider yourself to be?

[6] Definitely a morning type

[4] Rather more a morning type than an evening type

[2] Rather more an evening type than a morning type

[1] Definitely an evening type

_____ **Total points for all 19 questions**

Scoring *(We will come very shortly to what the different categories mean.)*

16–30	31–41	42–58	59–69	70–86
Definite evening	Moderate evening	Intermediate	Moderate morning	Definite morning

"RESEARCHERS HAVE GONE SO FAR AS TO SHOW THAT YOU CAN PREDICT WEIGHT LOSS SUCCESS BY MEASURING THE CIRCADIAN FLUCTUATIONS IN WRIST TEMPERATURE."

Another way to assess for your internal circadian rhythm is through wrist temperature. Sensors are available not only for research but also for anyone to buy online to assess their own rhythms. They are now in "smart watches" and some rings. In the case of a healthy circadian rhythm, your temperature should slowly rise during sleep, dropping slowly throughout the day until you go to sleep. There should be a slight bump in wrist temperature with meals, but otherwise the rhythm is smooth. Even if your circadian rhythm is disrupted for a short period of time, research shows that wrist temperature becomes erratic: it is not high enough at night and doesn't respond properly to food.[3] The curve is completely disrupted in those working night shift or those with irregular schedules.

Interestingly, our body temperature is also controlled by our circadian genes, so if you have a flat circadian rhythm, or your cycle is altered in its peaks and valleys, then you are at a similar metabolic risk to those who work night shifts. Researchers have gone so far as to show that you can predict weight loss success by measuring the circadian fluctuations in wrist temperature. Fascinating!

It was a powerful day when I realized how many of my patients who ate very late in the evening seemed to struggle to maintain their weight, or even keep on the plan that I outlined for them. This hit home for me when I had three women in one week who came in for different reasons, but all offered a similar initial story.

"RESEARCH HAS SHOWN THAT PEOPLE WHO ARE OF THE EVENINGNESS CIRCADIAN PATTERN HAVE A HIGHER LIKELIHOOD OF PUTTING ON WEIGHT AND MORE DIFFICULTY LOSING IT."

Raquel worked a job that kept her at work late at night, which is when she did her best work anyway. She would get home at 9:00 p.m., eat dinner at 10:00 p.m., and then snack until bedtime. She was not hungry in the morning, but could not help snacking throughout the day. Raquel wanted to lose 20 lbs, but she found that no matter what she did, those pounds were stuck to her midsection.

Geneviève, on the other hand, was trying to improve her diet to get pregnant. She was married to an Italian man, and ever since they were together she found herself eating late at night because that is when he was used to eating. She had not gained that much weight, but she noticed her weight had shifted to her stomach, her period had become more irregular, and she was always hungry, even right after a meal.

Melissa had always been heavier than she wanted and had always gained weight easily. She also found that she was able to drop the pounds with diet and exercise. That was, until she started taking night classes. She was so passionate about the art she was learning that she knew stress couldn't be involved. Melissa began to struggle to lose weight. Worse, she started to see her blood sugar rising, and she was feeling dizzy and irritable almost daily.

What did all of these women have in common? Well, they all identified themselves as night people, even scoring themselves as eveningness type on the circadian pattern questionnaire above, and they had newly adopted evening schedules.

Risks of Being a Nighttime Person

If, after taking the "Morningness-Eveningness Questionnaire," you just identified yourself as an eveningness type, or have an altered wrist temperature pattern, what does that say about you? Research has shown that people who are of the evening-ness circadian pattern have a higher likelihood of putting on weight and more dif-ficulty losing it.[5,6] That doesn't seem fair, now, does it? What generally happens is that you end up eating your meals in a period that your body has deemed as a time of rest. This alters how your body burns fat and also how it programs fat storage. When there is a disconnect between what you are doing and what your body thinks you should be doing, you will pack away all of the nutrients from a meal, whether it's healthy or unhealthy. In other words, you will gain far more weight than some-one who is eating in sync with their circadian rhythm, no matter what type of food you are eating.[5,6] Now that is some persuasive information!

We also know that people who have an eveningness type rhythm, or an altered circadian rhythm, tend to be more hungry, feel less satisfaction with meals, and also have less energy and motivation to exercise, or even move around throughout the day (the latter is a tendency formally known as *non-exercise activity thermogenesis*). Not only do these circadian rhythm changes have impacts on our ability to reach our aesthetic goals, but they can also make us feel sleepy and weepy all day long because of the impact on our physiology, which appears in various forms.

Oxidative Stress

Oxidative stress has been noted as one of the main forces behind heart disease, obesity, premature aging, autoimmune disease, fertility issues, cancer, and just about every other chronic disease. A visual example of this oxidative stress system at work is rust. When oxygen interacts with metal on your car, for example, the metal can change colour, become brittle, and fall apart. In the human body a disconnect occurs between the enzymes that create the (bad) oxidants, or free radicals, and the (good) antioxidants, that sweep them up. Part of the reason the disconnect occurs is that you need proper circadian signalling to tell your body when to make each of these. In the rust example, metal does not have antioxidants to protect it; therefore, when the damage occurs there is nothing in place to stop it or repair the broken metal. This is why antioxidants are so important! And you need to have a proper circadian cycle to make enough of them.

Reduction-Oxidation ("redox") reactions in your body are a natural process that allows you to use nutrients as fuel and then break down and eliminate the waste products from your digestion, metabolism, immune system, etc. A properly functioning redox system is also important to allow your cells to talk to each other, to fight cancer and infections. Even though we view free radicals as always bad, they do have very important functions, and we are continuously learning more and more about that function in health, weight loss, hormonal balance, and immune function. The issues arise when you're not eating well, your system is stressed out, and your circadian rhythm isn't timed properly. As with the rust example above, you have too much oxidation and not enough reduction if you have too many free radicals and not enough antioxidants. The result: more damage occurs than the body can keep up with. That is why I cover not only the circadian rhythms in this book, but why I will also address dietary antioxidants in upcoming chapters.

Health Consequences of Disrupted Circadian Rhythm
The more we study circadian rhythm issues, the more we discover about the power of these rhythms. For instance, 15% of all of our genetics are on a circadian pattern. Even if you are not a night-shift worker, but you are just a night owl or have an irregular eating time, these factors are enough to increase your risks for the following health concerns.

- Metabolic syndrome: includes obesity, type 2 diabetes, and high blood pressure, putting you at greater risk for cardiovascular disease as well
- Insulin resistance: includes weight loss resistance, hormonal imbalances, skin changes, and an increased risk of diabetes and heart disease
- Non-alcoholic fatty liver disease (NAFLD): includes insulin resistance, inflammation, and altered repair systems so that fat accumulates in the liver, and liver damage can result
- Increased oxidative stress: involves cellular damage and decreased cellular repair
- Cancer: oncologists use the power of circadian rhythms to treat cancer, as there are often circadian disruptions involved in the disease process[7]

Before we can explore how to get your circadian rhythm back on track, we need to look at the sorts of things that disrupt it. For example, if you eat the perfect meal at the wrong time of day, you may still struggle with weight loss resistance! Addressing the circadian rhythm first ensures that you will be able to see the full benefit of the strategies in the upcoming chapters.

"HOW OFTEN HAVE YOU DRIVEN HOME FROM WORK LATE AT NIGHT, OR SAT IN A DIMLY LIT ROOM TO RELAX, AND THEN AFTERWARDS YOU WENT TO HAVE A MEAL, OR EVEN A SNACK. THIS IS MASSIVELY DISRUPTIVE!"

What Disrupts Your Circadian Rhythm?

I am about to make a controversial statement, so keep an open mind and work with me here, okay? I do not believe that anyone is "naturally" a night owl. So many of my patients will say that they do their best work at night, and that's when they have the most energy. Although I do believe that's true for them, I also believe that it's a learned pattern, even if learned from a young age. How does one "learn" to disrupt their circadian rhythm?

Light exposure and unbalanced light-dark cycles are, in my opinion, the biggest disruptor of our circadian clock. When was the last time you were in true darkness? I mean no lights on, no phone, no TV, no street lights, no light pollution. For many of us it has been years, decades, or possibly never. I grew up camping, and I always say the forest is my happy place, the only place where I can truly slow my type A high-achieving mind and rest. This is true for many other women whom I have pretty much arm twisted into experiencing the true darkness of only star light. All of that light we are getting at night interacts with our brains to tell our bodies that it is daylight; therefore, those daytime bodily processes occur. These processes include increasing cortisol (your stress hormone), decreasing melatonin (your sleep hormone), increasing blood pressure, and decreasing the body's very important antioxidant and anti-inflammatory systems.[1,4]

One of the other main disruptors of your circadian rhythm is food intake.[5] How often have you driven home from work late at night, or sat in a dimly lit room to relax, and then afterwards you went to have a meal, or even a snack. This is massively disruptive! Just when your body is getting ready to wind down and go into cleanup mode (which happens as you sleep), you jump right back into food consumption and breakdown cycles. Your body gets confused and actually uncouples, or disconnects, your brain's circadian rhythm from the circadian rhythm of other tissues, like your fat cells and your liver—both of which are critical to attain your fat loss goals!

As I see more and more patients struggle to lose weight, I also see the evolution of circadian-disrupting technologies. I am not against technology by any means (hey, it's what allowed me to bring you this book!), but when you come to understand the power of how it can affect you in subtle but life-altering ways, I hope you will start to use technology's power for the good. You will learn how to do this throughout the chapter.

Optimal circadian rhythms

Before diving into how to repair the systems, let's take a quick review about what **should** happen during the biological daytime and what **should** happen during the biological nighttime. Remember, if your body is confused about whether it's daytime or nighttime by getting bright light at night for example, then the nighttime bodily functions don't happen efficiently. This is where many problems start!

Table 1. Summary of optimal circadian activities

Biological Daytime Events	Biological Nighttime Events
• Cortisol rises • Energy and alertness increase • Blood pressure increases • Metabolic hormones increase (determining fat burning or sugar burning)	• Melatonin increases • Immune system cleans up after a day's worth of waste • Antioxidants are produced • Metabolic storage hormones are low • Appetite and satiety hormones are regulated • Psychological repair occurs • Memory consolidation

Circadian Rhythm Repair

Even I fight to maintain a decent circadian rhythm, and I will not pretend it's easy. Everything and its mother wants to disrupt our cycles. That said, there are key things you can do to improve your rhythms, improve your health, and lose that stubborn weight (especially that belly fat) that I know you have been working so hard to lose.

Get Your Right Light On

Believe it or not, the main thing you need to consider when trying to get your circadian rhythm (and fat-burning metabolic rhythm) back on track is light exposure. The two most important factors include minimizing your artificial light at night and actually getting light in the morning. The invention of the light bulb was step one of the circadian disruption cycle. Think about it: without artificial light would you be up all hours eating, exercising, or watching TV? Not only does artificial light allow us to change the timing of our daily activities but also it disrupts our circadian rhythm.

Limit Night Light

When it comes to limiting light at night, I tend to be a realist, not a purist. I think it's critical to take a hard look at our technology use at night to do a night light inventory. (See the workbook at **www.sarahwilsonnd.com/loseitbookbonus.**) It is so easy for light to sneak in from unnecessary overhead lights, from your phone, tablet, television, and the like. All of these things blast out blue spectrum light.

Do you remember the ROYGBIV light spectrum from grade school? If not, there are multiple different spectrums of light, from warm light (red and orange), to cool light (blue and indigo). These different light spectrums also have different health effects and benefits. Red light is commonly researched to help with mental focus and potentially even mitochondrial health (the energy powerhouses). Green light has been said to stimulate our parasympathetic and digest and rest, nervous system. And blue light, well that is what we need to limit at night.

Blue light is the main circadian regulator. It is the light you want to limit from your electronic devices at night and what you want to increase in the morning to activate your morning processes and release cortisol to tell you when to wake up. My favourite app for controlling my light exposure is f.lux, which limits blue light exposure on devices such as computers and phones. Most phones now even have a blue-blocking screen setting (how cool!), which prevents some of the damaging circadian effects of after-sunset technology use. Other considerations include the light exposures in your bedroom. Do you have bright light streaming in from street lights? Or an obnoxiously bright alarm clock? We will chat about this further in the sleep section, but do what you can to limit these sources now.

Limiting nighttime light allows your body to define light/dark cycles, develop a period of hormonal reset and immune system cleanup, and regulate your hunger and fullness. Before we get too excited by the anti-aging, waistline trimming, energy-boosting effects of this strategy, we have to close the loop and signal morning to your body by getting morning light exposure.

"NOT COINCIDENTALLY, SEASONAL AFFECT DISORDER (OR SEASONAL DEPRESSION) AND WEIGHT GAIN ARE MORE COMMON IN THE WINTER MONTHS FOR MANY PEOPLE IN NORTHERN CLIMATES."

Maximize Morning Light

After spending the night asleep in darkness, it's important to get bright light in the morning to "retrain'" or reset your circadian rhythm. For those of you closer to the equator this is easier to achieve year-round as the sun's rays hit at a direct angle, and you have similar hours of light all year. Up here in good ol' Canada, and for many in the Northern United States, this isn't something we inherently count on in every season. Our hours of light exposure change from approximately nine hours in December to approximately fifteen hours in July. And given where we are situated, the sun's rays hit the earth at a different angle in the winter than they do in the summer. The combination of decreased natural light exposure and differing angles dictated by our geographic location has a huge impact on our circadian rhythms.

Not coincidentally, seasonal affect disorder (or seasonal depression) and weight gain are more common in the winter months for many people in northern climates. Although winter tends to be the time of many holiday celebrations, that alone does not account for all the weight changes we see in the winter. Some researchers believe that increased winter weight gain is partially related to circadian rhythm changes.[8] These alterations affect metabolic hormones, non-exercise activity thermogenesis, and cravings (hello, comfort foods!).

To counter these unwelcome effects, it is very important to get at least 20 minutes of bright light each morning. That may not sound like much, but if you live in a big city, it's quite possible to never see the light of day. For example, I have an underground garage at my home, as does my office building, and my gym. Even many grocery stores have them. It may be a vampire's dream come true, but before our inner Buffy gets too excited, think about the consequences. If your body does not get morning light exposure, then you won't have a strong "hey, its morning" signal. Your cortisol and digestive functions will be weak at best, and you can lose the sync and rhythm of your metabolic hormones. Research shows those who get proper morning light not only have improved moods and energy but also they have a lower body mass index, or weight.[9]

Take Action

Do not head for the next chapter before installing f.lux, closing your curtains at night, and maybe even buying a good old-fashioned paperback to read to limit the need to stare into light devices. These strategies will support your biological nighttime processes.

In the summer months, I like to get my morning light with a walk outside—with no sunglasses by the way. (Sunglasses by definition change the light that the eyes become exposed to.) This gets my blood moving and my eyes set to a morning light rhythm. On the dimmer winter mornings, I make use of my light box. I have the HappyLight, but there are many options. Turning this on while you put on your make-up, eat breakfast, or write in your journal (like I do) can be a great way to sync up without hampering your routine.

I have also used a dawn-stimulating alarm clock, which slowly brightens your dark room, signalling the time to get up, before your alarm sounds. Although most of these don't have the high flux, circadian resetting bright light, they can still be helpful to those who find themselves dragging in the morning.

"HEALTHY PEOPLE WHO EAT AFTER SUNDOWN HAVE THE SAME HORMONAL RESPONSE AS SOMEONE WITH TYPE 2 DIABETES!"

Meal Timing

Food has a way of telling your body what time it is. Just as light has effects on the brain, food intake changes the timing of "clocks" in the liver, pancreas, and kidneys. These are called *peripheral clocks*, and they send signals back to the brain to help coordinate the circadian cycle.[4,10] They dictate when to make digestive enzymes, when to make metabolic hormones (such as leptin, insulin, glucagon, and ghrelin to name a few), and also how much to make. As I've mentioned, research shows that when we alter eating patterns, when we eat irregularly or eat during the dark cycle of our circadian rhythm, these things can wreak havoc on our systems. In other words, eating every two hours or eating late at night has a significant effect on your level of insulin resistance, your fat loss potential, and even your feeling of fullness with meals. This means it's time to cut the snacking! Warning: what you are about to read may be contrary to some of what you have learned in all of your days of dieting.

Healthy people who eat after sundown have the same hormonal response as someone with type 2 diabetes! Yes, those with a healthy metabolism will have large elevations in both glucose and insulin, far beyond what they would experience if they ate the same food at lunch.[5] What does this mean? Well, insulin is a fat storage hormone, so that means your late-night snack goes right to your belly and stays there! Ideally, insulin should be low overnight and between meals to allow you to burn your fat as fuel.

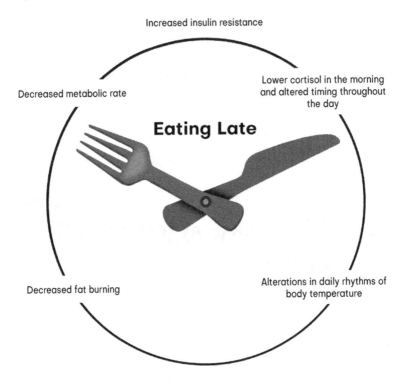

Figure 4. When you eat in your biological nighttime, your body isn't able to tolerate glucose, so your blood sugar and insulin rise. Altered rhythms with body temperature occur, impeding weight loss, and then how many calories your body burns at a baseline (your basal metabolic rate) decreases. Stress hormones are also affected so that you can feel exhausted and frazzled throughout the day.

I'm also commonly asked about timing coffee throughout the day. We don't know that coffee has a direct effect on the circadian rhythm, but it has a dramatic impact on sleep. We will explore the effects of coffee in **chapter 3**, but for now try to keep your java to the morning hours, and definitely before 2:00 p.m.

Take Action

We'll get into the science of the snack in **chapter 6**, and I promise that I'll put this all together for you in a feeling awesome, fat-burning-machine kind of day at the end of this book. In the meantime, your action for today is simply to limit your eating cycle to sun-up hours. Depending on the time of year and your location, those hours will fluctuate slightly. Consult your local weather network to check times for sunrise and sunset. Then eat within these hours. (Hint: be realistic with yourself here. If you are not the type of person to check in with the sun's waking hours regularly, then just set a time for yourself, i.e., no eating between 7:00 p.m. and 7:00 a.m.)

The Exercise Factor

It has been shown that movement patterns throughout the day are both affected by and affect circadian rhythms. However, there is little research to suggest that weight loss resistance or metabolic syndrome are improved by exercising at one specific time or another. My recommendation on timing is to avoid high-intensity workouts after 6:00 p.m. After this hour, high-intensity exercise can change your stress hormone production and also prevent you from getting to sleep on time.

If you have struggled with weight loss programs before, feel like you can't stay on a plan, or just aren't losing weight, which is most of us—that's why you're here, right?—the circadian rhythm steps laid out above are a *must*! Even if it doesn't feel natural at first, push yourself to get on track with your circadian rhythm. It's easier than giving up chocolate as a first step, isn't it?

Take Action

Be realistic. Don't aim to wake a 6:00 a.m. to work out if you aren't a morning person, yet. And don't try to go to spinning classes five times a week if you haven't been to the gym in years. Start by moving your body, preferably in the morning so you know it's done, in ways that are enjoyable for you and that fit into your schedule.

Working the Night Shift?

What do you do if—like Kennedy—you have to go to work at night? The key is maintaining a degree of consistency. If your days are split fifty-fifty, nights versus days, then you will need to find a happy medium.

For many of my patients that means on their night-shift days they have a really large "breakfast," which would be our dinner, and then they eat again just as the sun is starting to come up. This skips snacking and eating during the biological nighttime.

Blue-blocking glasses or lenses can be helpful to minimize the effects of blue light on the circadian rhythm. It's also critical to sleep in complete, blackout darkness on those night shifts and on the mornings that you are not working to use light boxes to reset the circadian cycle.

Finally, supplementation is often necessary. Adaptogens, herbs I discuss in **chapter 4**, can be incredibly helpful to support cortisol rhythms and energy levels throughout the day/night. At times, very low-dose melatonin, the sleep hormone, can be used to help your body maintain a nighttime, even if you are working. However, this is a case by case basis as melatonin makes some people much sleepier than others.

Overall, do the best you can to implement the advice in this chapter, and the other information in this book that is pertinent for you. It is most often enough to help you overcome your plateaus. If not, seek out a naturopathic doctor who is comfortable with the treatment of this area for further support.

Are you wondering what happened for the patients I've discussed so far? Not only did they lose weight but they also improved their energy, skin, mood, and digestion. Kennedy actually ended up changing her job based on the information she learned and has made it a priority to use this information to educate her fellow nurses on how to keep healthy on night duty shifts. Raquel's success started with blue blockers and light boxes. Within four nights of using blue-blocking glasses, she felt like she slept more soundly. When we started working together, it was the dead of winter so the light box provided a much-needed morning energy boost. What Raquel didn't expect was that her cravings would also decrease, and going longer without snacks became easy. It took a full two weeks on the plan before Raquel started to see any weight loss (in hindsight, she said the mindset pieces were the only things keeping her going). Thank goodness she pushed through the discomfort though, as Raquel lost on average two pounds per week after that and has been able to maintain her goal weight.

Genevieve got pregnant and is now dealing with a whole new kind of circadian disruption (a nursing baby!). Melissa restricted her eating window, got an extra hour of sleep, and found her blood sugar regulation completely changed. For her, the sleep was almost as important to her weight loss as the circadian rhythm changes. Which is what we'll be diving into next. It's the sleep–wake cycle after all, so let's find out how your sleep could be locking your fat-burning mode!

The Finally Lose It Circadian Review

- Your circadian rhythm is a twenty-four-hour clock that determines your hormonal response, inflammation levels, sleep and wake cycles, and digestive function.
- The main disruptors of the circadian rhythm are blue light at night, and conversely no light in the morning, and also eating at irregular times or in your biological night.
- A disrupted circadian rhythm has been associated with cardiovascular disease, diabetes, insulin resistance, premature aging, insomnia, weight loss resistance, and even cancer.
- Your morningness and eveningness circadian rhythm type can be determined by the questionnaire above. Researchers have shown that those with an eveningness chronotype are less likely to lose weight, stick with a change, and if they do lose weight are more likely to gain it back.
- Changing the type and timing of your light exposure and eating at set times that occur during your biological daytime are critical for the balance of your circadian rhythm.

SLEEP IS THE GOLDEN CHAIN THAT TIES HEALTH AND OUR BODIES TOGETHER.

—THOMAS DEKKER

without having to snack all day. Becky lost four dress sizes in a way that she never imagined possible: with eventual ease, self-love, and through nourishing herself—all in three months' time!

When it comes to control of our metabolism and hormones, we do not talk enough about sleep. Most of us associate need for sleep with fatigue, with that fried and easily irritated feeling, but how often do we sit back and think to ourselves, *hmmm, I bet I could sleep away these 20 lbs*. Likely never! But sleep is incredibly important to weight loss. Although we each have individual sleep requirements, research shows that people who sleep less than seven hours per night have a 30% increased risk of being obese.[11] You read that correctly! If I asked you to decrease your risk of obesity by 30%, you would jump at the chance I bet. So here is your invitation to do just that.

What Happens During Sleep?

First, let's explore what exactly sleep is and why we talk about it as this elusive state. We truly have no idea why we sleep. We can go from being fully conscious and present in our lives to unconscious in a matter of minutes! There is good reason for sleep as we will see, but we will never know the full extent of what happens during this period or why we need it.

DID YOU KNOW THAT WE (SHOULD) SLEEP FOR A TOTAL OF ONE-THIRD OF OUR LIVES?

We have two main categories of sleep: non-rapid eye movement (NREM) and rapid eye movement (REM). We cycle through four stages of NREM sleep and REM sleep throughout the night. REM sleep is most notably characterized by increased nervous system activity, dream-related sleep, and memory consolidation. NREM sleep, on the other hand, is often associated with growth hormone production. In addition to growth hormone manufacture, your sleep also dictates the patterns of cortisol release, thyroid hormone production, and leptin (your fat stat) and ghrelin (your hunger hormone) production.[12,13] I bet you're starting to better appreciate just how busy our bodies are while we sleep.

Sleep Stages

Stage 1	Stage 2	Stage 3	Stage 4	Stage 5
· Light sleep. · Muscle activity slows down. · Occasional muscle twitching. · Growth hormone released.	· Breathing pattern and heart rate slow. · Slight decrease in body temperature. · Brain generates spindle waves.	· Deep sleep begins. · Brain begins to generate slow delta waves.	· Very deep sleep. · Rhythmic breathing. · Limited muscle activity. · Brain produces delta waves.	· Rapid eye movement (REM Sleep.) · Brainwaves speed up and dreaming occurs. · Muscles relax and heart rate increases. · Breathing is rapid and shallow.

Figure 5. Sleep is a critical time for your body to clean up inflammation, regulate its hormone release, rest, and repair. Deep sleep periods are required for proper growth hormone release, leptin and ghrelin release, appetite control, and control of the circadian rhythm.

As you might imagine, for deep and restful sleep to occur your body should be downregulating the stress response, including lowering cortisol, and the fight or flight hormones norepinephrine and epinephrine. The lowering of these levels should coincide with an increase in melatonin, which is one of the hormones involved in sleep onset and maintenance.

In addition to these hormonal changes, sleep is critically important for your immune system. During sleep, your immune system revs up, clearing out the junk your body has accumulated throughout the day.[14,15] It also takes stock of the viruses and infections you fought that day so that your body knows what to do when it sees them next. During sleep, your body also begins to increase the activity of regulatory

T cells.[16] These bad boys control the body's immune system, keeping inflammation and autoimmune disease in check; they are essential to long-term health. The anti-aging movement has been invested in sleep research for many years, as we know that oxidative stress—one of the major factors involved in aging—is kept under control during sleep. Did you know that we (should) sleep for a total of one-third of our lives?

"WHEN YOU ARE NOT SLEEPING WELL, NOT LONG ENOUGH, NOT DEEP ENOUGH, AT THE WRONG HOURS, OR WHEN YOUR SLEEP IS DISRUPTED, THAT IS WHEN THE PROVERBIAL SHIT JUST HITS THE FAN"

Of course, in order for all the magic of the human sleep cycle to happen, we need to be asleep! Not just for a few hours, but for more than seven and a half. Those hours of sleep can't just be from 4:00 a.m. to 12:00 p.m. either. When it comes to sleep, timing and duration are everything. When you are not sleeping enough, you do not spend enough time in each sleep cycle, and the benefits of each cycle are simply not seen. In order to get the full benefits, you need to get your butt in bed by 11:00 p.m. at the latest. This is where the circadian rhythm and sleep intersect in a crucial way. We are programmed to do our best sleep work from approximately 11:00 p.m. to 4:00 a.m. When you are not sleeping well, not long enough, not deep enough, at the wrong hours, or when your sleep is disrupted, that is when the proverbial shit just hits the fan.[14]

Why Sleep Eludes You

Now that I have convinced you that you need more sleep and you are 100% on board and just can't wait to experience the full benefits of a night of restful, metabolism-boosting, immune-calming, brain-cleansing sleep, let's address the elephant in the room: insomnia. You may be thinking, this is well and good for Becky, now that all she has to do is take more time to sleep, but I can't freaking sleep!

You are not alone. One in three North Americans experience insomnia in their lifetime, and women are twice as likely as men to experience sleep disturbances. I would say that around 50% of the women in my practice experience difficulty falling asleep with or without racing thoughts, waking throughout the night to pee, or waking between 2:00 a.m and 4:00 a.m. reproducibly. Each of these pieces of information is important to consider and each one tells us about the other systems in your body, such as cortisol and insulin and blood sugar regulation.

The reality is that only about 5% of the population qualifies as short sleepers, meaning that, for whatever reason, they are able to stay metabolically healthy in the face of a short sleep cycle. As much as we may pretend we are in that percentage, we most likely are not. Heck, maybe that's what has brought you here. Sleep may be "the thing" that is preventing you from achieving your health goals. This was certainly true for Becky. Let's take a closer look at the many influences on compromised sleep.

"MELATONIN IS A VERY STRONG ANTIOXIDANT, IN ADDITION TO ITS ROLE IN SLEEP ONSET, AND WHAT WE ARE COMING TO KNOW IS THAT WITHOUT ANTIOXIDANTS, OXIDATIVE STRESS CAN NEGATIVELY IMPACT YOUR IMMUNE SYSTEM, METABOLISM, SEX HORMONES, YOUR MOOD, AND MEMORY"

Melatonin and Cortisol

Melatonin, the hormone associated with sleep and nighttime, promotes relaxation and is only released in the darkness. Melatonin is highly sensitive, I mean "man with the flu" sensitive. Melatonin production will decrease with any bright light exposure, especially blue lights from florescent light bulbs, phones, and TV screens. When we have a decrease in our melatonin production, we can also have an increase in cortisol. These two hormones function like a teeter-totter, when one end is high, the other is low. When cortisol is elevated after a stressful day at work, a fight with a partner, or from blue light exposure, you may not only struggle to get to sleep, but we also have a lower quality of restorative sleep. The reason is that melatonin is a very strong antioxidant, in addition to its role in sleep onset, and what we are coming to know is that without antioxidants, oxidative stress can negatively impact your immune system, metabolism, sex hormones, mood, and memory.[13,17]

Cortisol Awakening Response and Blood Sugar Dysregulation

In addition to the effects of cortisol keeping your mind racing at night because of its suppression of melatonin, we also have a pattern in our bodies known as the cortisol awakening response (CAR). This is exactly what it sounds like: cortisol is not all bad in the body, and it should naturally start to rise in the morning to wake us up, all bright-eyed and bushy-tailed. When things are working well in our bodies, this awakening should happen between 6:00 a.m. and 7:00 a.m. But with chronic stress, things go awry.

Have you ever woken between 2:00 a.m. and 4:00 a.m. and felt wide awake? Some of you may experience it as a revved-up, spring out of bed feeling, whereas others will wake and then find they just lay there for hours with their mind wandering. These cases are very common with low cortisol levels or a dysregulated CAR. I remember in my first year of medical school, 2:42 a.m. and I had a very close relationship; in fact, we met just about every morning until I started to manage my cortisol response. Many of you will have similar stories.

The 2:00–4:00 a.m. awakening is a red flag for stress, cortisol and blood sugar dysregulation. You may think that you don't feel overly stressed, so that waking through the night must be for a different reason. And you may be mistaken. Although blood sugar dysregulation is not a typical type of stress, your body still has to use cortisol to correct it. Indeed, you need to have a pretty healthy metabolic hormone system in order to regulate your blood glucose overnight. You should ideally keep your glucose level between 4.7 and 5.0 mmol/L (85 and 90 mg/dl) so that your brain has fuel to keep you alive. When this does not happen because of issues with insulin sensitivity, growth hormone, or inflammation, you have to use cortisol to increase blood sugar levels to fuel the brain. This cortisol spike that happens can also result in you waking up during the night. We will dive into strategies to solve this issue below and in **chapter 4**, but if you are in this boat, mark this page, because what you are about to learn can change your life!

Anxiety

If your mind is continuously racing when you are trying to fall asleep, if you find you are worrying or replaying the negative events of the day over and over, then you are like the many women who visit my office. Let's be real for a moment: most of us have experienced anxiety to some degree or other. I cannot tell you how many times I have laid in bed at night thinking about all the things that I didn't get done, all the patients that need follow-up, and all the articles, books, videos that I want to get done. And that's not even the personal stuff! I would argue that next to cortisol and blood sugar, anxiety is there among the biggest triggers perpetuating the cycle of poor sleep and more belly fat.

In the face of anxiety, it is not only the effects on sleep that can lead to weight gain, but also the hormonal environment changes. With anxiety, cortisol, norepinephrine, and epinephrine often surge throughout the day. This affects blood sugar but it also affects your ability to use fat as fuel. When you are stuck in sugar-burning mode, it can also affect your sleep because you may wake up in the middle of the night starving for something to give your body enough energy to continue on. A bit of a double whammy here, I would say! You can lose sleep at the outset as racing thoughts keep you from falling asleep and then you wake up, losing more sleep and disrupting all of that hormone-balancing, inflammation-decreasing sleepy goodness. (Before moving forward I want to note that the solution to significant anxiety may not be in this book. The principles in this and other chapters may help, but don't hesitate to seek other resources to support you if you feel anxiety is a main factor for you.)

Progesterone

Progesterone may just be my favourite female sex hormone because it is calming, anti-inflammatory, and, to be honest, helps to keep my mood and my relationships stable! It is also one of the most coveted hormones in the female reproductive cycle: have you ever wished that your PMS symptoms would decrease, your period cramps or heavy flow would vanish, or yearned for more restorative sleep? If you say yes to any of the above, then you have experienced a craving for progesterone.

Progesterone acts directly on the sleep centres of the brain, helping to calm you into sleep. Additionally, progesterone is able to influence certain neurotransmitters, specifically gamma-Aminobutyric acid (GABA) and serotonin. GABA is a calming neurotransmitter, and serotonin has been known as the "happy hormone," so you can imagine how they would affect restorative sleep. Sleep studies have also shown that when progesterone is highest during the last two weeks before your period we also see more sleep spindles, indicating a deeper sleep.[18]

Low levels of progesterone are not only the plague of the modern menstruating woman but they are also at play in the sleep issues that come with menopause. So if you feel as if you aren't able to calm down properly into sleep, you have light or broken sleep, and you do not identify with any of the other factors listed here, it may be time to check those hormones.

Sleep Apnea

Sleep apnea, the unsung villain of sleep disturbance, is a condition in which people experience interrupted breathing throughout the night. Untreated sleep apnea can lead to low oxygen levels to the brain and other tissues, which results in long-term serious health consequences, and it also affects sleep quality and metabolic hormonal balance. Many people do not know they are suffering from sleep apnea until they have a sleep study, because many of the symptoms are considered "normal." Some signs you might notice if you have sleep apnea include loud snoring, restless sleep, waking with a headache or dry irritated throat, unrefreshing sleep, sleepiness during the day, and forgetfulness or poor memory. If you have any of these, or if you find you wake at night gasping for air, then do yourself a favour and get to a sleep clinic. Adequate oxygen can save your waistline but, more importantly, your life!

Caffeine Hygiene

I have banged my head countless times against the wall trying to figure out why a patient is struggling with sleep, only to find that they are having coffee late in the afternoon or with dinner. Now believe me, I love coffee as much as you do. There is nothing quite like that cup of joe in the morning or after lunch to put a smile on your face and a pep in your step! (It is also a nice excuse to get up from your desk.)

Logic tells us that coffee is not sleep's friend. The caffeine in coffee will increase epinephrine, your fight or flight stress system, which takes you right out of that melatonin-producing, rest and relax mode so critical for quality sleep. Here's what you may not know: caffeine doesn't just affect you while you are drinking it. In fact, it can take between three and seven hours for the caffeine to break down. This time frame depends on your health, liver function, genetics, digestion, and hormonal balance. I, for example, am genetically a slow metabolizer. So for me, there's no caffeine after 2:00 p.m. Some people can have coffee after dinner and still sleep like a baby, but that's rare! If sleep is a struggle, make sure one of the first things you check is the timing of your caffeine intake.

"SOME STUDIES HAVE SHOWN THAT WITH ONLY A FEW DAYS OF SLEEP RESTRICTION YOU CAN SEE A 40% DECREASE IN GLUCOSE TOLERANCE! THAT MEANS THAT IF YOU HAD A PIECE OF CHOCOLATE WITH 20 G OF SUGAR IN IT, YOUR BODY WOULD RESPOND AS IF YOU HAD EATEN ALMOST 35 G."

When Sleep Is Lacking, Fat Loss Goes Packing

Sleep reduction can quickly leave you in a brain foggy, hangry, fat-storing, sugar-burning state. We've considered the reasons that sleep may be eluding you. Now it's time to explore the effects of reduced sleep and to see what might resonate most strongly with your experience.

Glucose and Insulin

Just as issues with circadian rhythmicity affect insulin and glucose levels, changes to sleep can also affect insulin and glucose levels within days. Some studies have shown that with only a few days of sleep restriction you can see a 40% decrease in glucose tolerance. That means that if you had a piece of chocolate with 20 g of sugar in it, your body would respond as if you had eaten almost 35 g.[19] Results have also suggested a 30% decrease in insulin responsiveness. Therefore, in *healthy* people, with less than one week of four hours' sleep per night, their blood sugar was higher and they were more insulin resistant, to the point that they appeared to be pre-diabetic!

You aren't entirely out of the woods if you are getting more than four hours of sleep but still less than seven. Another study looking at subjects sleeping seven to eight and a half hours versus less than six and a half hours, found that those in the latter category may not have had a drastic change in their glucose levels, but they still had an increase in circulating insulin by 50% and experienced a 40% decrease in insulin sensitivity. In terms of weight loss resistance, these increases are significant.

These changes will lock your fat stores away in the deep freeze, preventing you from efficiently using fat as fuel, which works against your belly fat–burning goals. We'll explore the details further in **chapter 6.**

Leptin

On those (now rare) days when I am sleep-deprived, the drive toward high-fat, high-sugar foods is at its strongest. Have you ever wondered why so many breakfast foods are sugar laden, carbohydrate dense, and often fat filled? Foods such as bagels with cream cheese, toast and peanut butter, and, heaven forbid, deep-fried hash browns or eggs with cheese on English muffins permeate our breakfast culture. It's no coincidence that the lineup at your local breakfast place on a Friday morning has grown in tandem with the rates of sleep deprivation. Some people argue that the drive toward these foods is due to a lack of time to prepare breakfast, but I suggest that your leptin and ghrelin are responsible for those choices as well.

When I first heard about leptin, I was working in an obesity research lab. In our department, there were discussions about appetite, satiety, and the self-regulation of fat cells through something called *adipocytokines* (messages sent by our fat cells). We were realizing that fat, once thought to be this glob of useless cells, was actually an endocrine tissue, communicating its state and needs to the rest of the body. One of the signals that these fat cells would send was leptin.

Leptin's role is to communicate to the brain how much fat we have. The more fat, the more overweight we are, the more leptin circulating. Leptin signals your brain, "Okay body, we need to get rid of some of this stuff," and it increases the basal metabolic rate (metabolism), it increases your drive to move your body (fidgeting, walking, keeping active outside of exercise), and it also decreases your appetite. It is a brilliant system when you think about it. We really thought we were on to something in the research community with the finding that some people who were morbidly obese from a very young age were actually born with an error preventing them from making leptin. When these people were injected with leptin they naturally lost weight. Eureka! Let's just inject obese people with leptin to bring their weight into a healthy range.

As with everything in life, it wasn't that simple. It was quickly discovered that many obese people actually make an ample quantity of leptin, but as with insulin, when you make too much, your body just stops listening to the signal and becomes resistant. In these cases, we see that many people who struggle with their weight actually respond as if they need to conserve energy, move less, and eat more—they respond as if they have low levels of leptin.

You're probably wondering how this relates to our sleep. The control of leptin release occurs while we sleep. You can predict this isn't going to end well. Even with moderate sleep-time reduction, we see a drop in leptin up to 20%![20] This can result in your brain thinking that your body is carrying less fat than it is and thus decreasing your metabolism to protect you.

Ghrelin

A drop in leptin is also combined with an increase in ghrelin levels, which results in a double hit to your hunger and craving levels. Ghrelin, made primarily in the stomach, increases your appetite and your cravings. Ghrelin signals the brain that it's time to forage for food. I don't think any of us want to feel artificially hungry (starving, even) after just having a meal a few hours before, but this is what happens with sleep deprivation. We end up walking around with 25% more ghrelin than our well-slept neighbours. These cravings generally result in caving in, or using up all of your willpower by the end of the day, so that you fall face first into the chocolate cake at night. Imagine what it would be like to be 25% less hungry and have 25% fewer cravings.[11,20]

The effects of these hormones, although not always as apparent as I make them sound, can be significant. Just fighting off hunger, debating with snacking signals, or dealing with a slightly slower metabolism can seriously limit the enjoyment and success in your mission for health. Both leptin and ghrelin have been implicated in obesity and eating disorders, so the fact that you could sleep more and regulate these bad boys is key information.

Growth Hormone

As its name suggests, growth hormone is a beautiful building hormone known to increase muscle, increase the metabolic rate, counteract the effects of insulin on the body, and keep us feeling and looking young and limber. What is critical to know at this juncture is that growth hormone is produced mainly in the slow wave cycles of sleep. Indeed, we have to be sleeping in order to get proper growth hormone release and in order to see the *counter regulatory* benefits. In other words, growth hormone is stimulating growth and the breakdown of fat in order to fuel that growth. This opposes insulin's action in fat storage. With a lack of sleep and thus a lack of growth hormone, you can see a gradually expanding waistline, diminishing strength, and premature aging.

Decision Fatigue

Picture this: all day long people have been asking you what to do, where to go, and how to get there. You come home on a Friday night after a long week with little sleep, and your partner asks what's for dinner. You throw up your hands, so done with having to decide things, and somehow end up at the pizza place around the corner. After eating, you ask yourself how on earth that happened, given that you're trying to make "better choices." This is decision fatigue. It's just what it sounds like, exhaustion from making decisions, and it's common with sleep deprivation. We are all the more susceptible because of craving comfort foods and the increased leptin and ghrelin activity. If your partner had said, "Let's go for salad," you probably would have ended up there instead. There is nothing quite like a lack of sleep to intensify your decision fatigue and mess with your ability to make and stick to a plan. This is why we have accountability partners: your fried-food-loving friend is not the person to hang out with on a Friday afternoon, your support partner is!

"PEOPLE ARE WILLING TO PAY MILLIONS OF DOLLARS FOR ANTI-AGING MEDICINES, SURGERIES, SUPPLEMENTS, AND PHARMACEUTICAL MEDICATIONS. THE GOAL HERE? AT THE END OF THE DAY WE ARE ALL MOTIVATED TO HAVE MORE ENERGY, LOOK MORE YOUTHFUL, HAVE BETTER ATTENTION AND FOCUS, AND LIVE IN A STATE OF CRAVINGS-FREE BLISS."

Movement and Exercise

When you are lacking sleep, you are also lacking energy to exercise. This connection seems obvious on the surface. Exercise is just one form of calorie-burning movement that occurs throughout our day, and frankly it makes up a very small portion of the energy we use in a day. Think about it: you are in the gym maybe one hour, three to four times per week (on a good week!). So that would be four out of 168 hours or 0.02% of your time. I am not suggesting that exercise is unimportant.

On the contrary, it has massive and long-lasting hormonal benefits. But it does mean that you should be able to lose weight without setting up camp at the gym.

One of the things that I encourage with patients is movement, known in the research as non-exercise activity thermogenesis (NEAT). NEAT makes up about 50% of the calories an active person uses and 6–10% of the calories a sedentary person burns throughout the day. NEAT includes things like standing, fidgeting, moving around the office or house, chopping, cooking, picking things up, etc. These are the activities of daily life that we often don't pay attention to.

When we are sleep-deprived, the fact that we do these activities subconsciously can actually work against us because we don't notice when we are *not* doing them. With sleep loss there is less movement and activity throughout the day, which can be a huge hindrance to our progress. Can you imagine eating 40% more calories throughout the day? Of course you would gain weight. Well, going from an active person with NEAT resulting in 50% of your calorie burn to sitting around all day and having NEAT at 10% of the energy used is similar in theory.[21] There are many researchers now investigating whether NEAT is involved with the current obesity epidemic.[22] The moral is, when we are not sleeping enough, we do not want to move, period.

Improve Your Sleep, Change Your Reality

The power of sleep in this program cannot be underestimated! People are willing to pay millions of dollars for anti-aging medicines, surgeries, supplements, and pharmaceutical medications. The goal here? At the end of the day we are all motivated to have more energy, look more youthful, have better attention and focus, and live in a state of cravings-free bliss. Admittedly, sleep alone may not give you that, but it is surely an important element to reaching these goals! Here are some strategies to help you meet that end.

Sleep Hygiene

Just as we explored nighttime circadian rhythm routines, we need to consider bedtime routines. We've established that limiting blue light exposure, shutting off screens at least an hour before bed, and sleeping in a pitch-black room are critical. Among the other practices to consider, your bedroom needs to be a cool temperature. One of the triggers for sleep onset is actually a drop in our body temperature. This is why for some people with insomnia or for kids, taking a warm bath and then jumping into bed can help initiate sleep. As your body cools down in the right environment, it signals sleeping time has arrived. If your room is too warm though, that drop in body temperature is blunted, and the signals for sleep can be thwarted as well.

Another practice critical to sleep hygiene is setting a consistent bedtime. For some of you that will mean setting a sleep-time alarm on your phone. When that alarm goes off, it should signal you to get your butt ready for bed, maybe do a bit of reading in a dimly lit room, and then off to sleep. The bedroom should also be reserved for sleep and sex only. Starting a fight with a partner? Watching a captivating show? Get out of that bedroom! When you are trying to fall asleep, that rise in energy is the last thing you need.

"AS A NATUROPATHIC DOCTOR I AM ALL ABOUT TREATING THE ROOT CAUSE AND GETTING TO THE BOTTOM OF CHRONIC CONDITIONS. FRANKLY, SUPPLEMENTS CAN HELP IN THIS, BUT LIFESTYLE CHANGES ARE GOLD!"

To-Do Journal

Have you ever jumped into bed only to have a thousand things that need to get done start to swirl around in your mind? Or maybe you're overcome with what feels like a thousand worries popping into your head at once. Night-before to-do journaling has worked wonders for my sleep quality. This activity, also called idea journaling or worry journaling, is exactly what it sounds like.

I have a journal beside my bed at all times, and on nights when I am feeling particularly overwhelmed, I will dive in and write things out. I recommend this strategy to make lists about the things that need to get done, to jot down ideas, and keep track of things that you don't want to forget. One of my patients, Susan, used hers specifically as a worry journal: she wrote about anything that popped into her head for 10 minutes before getting into bed every night. She told me that toward the end of her second week of doing this, she was able to laugh at some of her worries and push them aside. This helped Susan get to sleep and stay asleep better than any supplement ever had. I am in awe of the power of some of these activities, and so are my patients.

Yoga, Stretching, and Movement

If a racing mind, tightness, and tossing and turning seem to be involved with your sleep disturbances, then a bedtime yoga or stretching routine may be just the thing for you. Often getting into bed is the first moment of our day that we allow our minds to slow, trying to stop the onslaught of information that hits us throughout the day. This can be a dramatic change of pace for the body though, and a difficult transition from busyness to stillness. In these situations, I love combining movement with mindfulness before bed. I often use stretching, yoga, and slow movements as moving meditations. These are a great way to get in touch with your body, calm your mind, and centre yourself for the evening. The key to these activities is that they must be restful and relaxing. No power yoga or workout style yoga here please! What I often recommend are bedtime yoga sequences or videos, or listening to a meditation while stretching.

As a naturopathic doctor I am all about treating the root cause and getting to the bottom of chronic conditions. Frankly, supplements can help in this, but lifestyle changes are gold! If you have worked your way through some of the activities above and still aren't getting where you want to go, this is where we bring in the big guns.

Low-Dose Melatonin

You'll recall that melatonin is the sleep onset hormone. And as a hormone, we should not be using it as haphazardly as the current market is. In my opinion, if all you have is a sleep onset concern, there is no need for the 10–20 mg that some products recommend. As little as 1 mg of melatonin has been shown to increase sleep onset, and prolonged-release doses can help to keep you asleep.[23] Studies of 5 mg doses of melatonin show that this dose helps to improve your sleep quality, and some studies show a decrease in body mass index (BMI) in overweight women after 16 weeks of use. This was with no other changes to diet and lifestyle![17]

Although the dream of weight loss while you sleep may suddenly seem within reach, don't jump right into the 5 mg dose. With melatonin, you want to start low and increase slowly. Not only can you have the hangover drowsiness the next day, but melatonin can also cause very vivid dreams, which can actually waken people from sleep. (As with all the supplements in this book, if you are on other medications or living with a chronic disease then check with your medical practitioner before starting a new supplement regime.)

Magnesium

Due to our current food supply and all of the stressors that our bodies experience, magnesium is one of the most deficient minerals. It is too bad that most women don't know this because it can have a nice, relaxing effect on the body and the mind.

Many find that magnesium can be a very gentle sleep support, more facilitating sleep than pushing you into drowsiness. Magnesium also offers side benefits and has a good safety profile. Magnesium can help to decrease muscle tension, period cramps, headaches, and even help with sugar cravings. There are many different forms of magnesium, but each of them can contribute to diarrhea if taken at high doses. Magnesium glycinate or bisglycinate is a great form for sleep, having less bowel-loosening effects. Whichever you can find, studies show doses of 250–350 mg can be helpful to increase slow wave sleep, lower nighttime cortisol levels, and even lower inflammation, all while helping you to feel more rested![24,25] It comes in both capsule and powder form and can be taken before bed to help with sleep.

VSP

VSP is the abbreviated name of an herbal formula with valerian, skullcap, and passionflower. This herbal combination can work wonders when it comes to sleep and restfulness!

Valerian is calming, but I like to warn people before discussing its properties that it's uniquely smelly. If you are sensitive to the smell of old gym socks, say, then valerian might not be the choice for you. However, I think when something is powerful and effective, it's worth the smell, which becomes almost endearing over time (try to trust me here). Valerian's odour is as powerful as its ability to decrease anxiety, panic attacks, and tension in the body. Valerian has been used historically for sleep but also for stomach pain and tension headaches that affect sleep.

Skullcap, which is an awful name, is also known as *scutellaria lateriflora*. Skullcap has been used for centuries to ease irritability, emotional stress, premenstrual syndrome, and insomnia. It can also be incredibly helpful with nervous fatigue. Have you ever had a stressful day when you came home, fell on the couch, completely exhausted, and then when it was time for bed you were counting sheep? Welcome to nervous exhaustion; skullcap will definitely be your friend in these cases.

Passionflower's main indication is for nervousness, anxiety, or excitability that is taking away from falling asleep and staying asleep. I love passionflower tinctures as well when I just can't seem to calm myself or take the rev out of the engine, so to speak.

Although VSP usually comes together as a tincture with the three herbs because it works as a lovely trio, you can also buy them separately. When you are taking the combination, it's best to take 30 to 60 drops one hour before you hope to be asleep.

Sleepy Teas

Not everyone needs a powerful hit to their sleep systems. I have a lot of patients who are very sensitive to supplementation and need a gentle nudge as opposed to a push. In these cases, I love the sleepy tea formulations. I often use teas to help me sleep when I am excited or nervous about an event, a speaking gig, or something that is going to happen the next day. I can say that now because I have amazing sleep quality, but even when I was younger I would use these teas regularly to help overcome anxious thoughts and what I call "inflammatory worry," where I would have racing thoughts and an active brain, although no real worries.

My favourite herbal formulations for myself and my patients will have lemongrass, chamomile, tilia, lavender, or even California poppy. The other thing I like about these calming teas is that they are readily accessible. If you are having trouble with sleep onset then you could likely pop into your local grocery story or health food store and pick up something to try tonight. It's a great way to rest, relax, and ease your way into the evening, all while using the sedating properties of the herbs to help you get to sleep and stay asleep.

To prepare the tea use 1 bag, or 1 tsp. of dried herb in 1 cup of water. Steep, covered, for 10–15 minutes, and then enjoy. Bonus points if you enjoy your beverage in a lavender Epsom salts bath while reading this book!

Take Action

We all have a different tolerance for sleep reduction. Some people need as few as six hours, whereas others need eight to 10 hours. I find for most people, the sweet spot lies at seven to eight hours. Too much more and they get a sleep hangover, too little, and all the issues that Becky experienced, above, can arise. In either case, be honest with yourself about the sleep you need.

Look at why you are not sleeping as much:

- What are you doing during the hours you are not sleeping?
- What is your bedtime routine?
- How many hours of artificial light, blue light, are you getting before bed?
- Is there something in your life affecting your sleep? (Does your partner snore? Do you snore? Do you have sleep apnea? How dark is your room? What temperature is your room?)

Take a moment to write your responses down in your workbook (see **www.sarahwilsonnd.com/loseitbookbonus**) Understanding these aspects and improving upon them, even by 10% per night, can help you to lose weight effortlessly, not to mention improve your overall health, interactions, and energy throughout the day.

Years ago, when I checked in with myself and got honest about the sleep I needed (which is seven and half to nine hours, depending on the night), I realized how much needed to change. I was caught in a loop of chronic inflammation, insomnia, and blood sugar swings that first needed to be addressed before I was even able to sleep. When those concerns fell into place I felt my "willpower muscle" increase. I was able to eat intuitively for the first time, and my baseline stress and feelings of anxiety throughout the day decreased significantly. This will happen for you as well! Weight loss feels easy when you are not getting accidental calories, craving comfort foods, and feeling like a couch potato.

The Finally Lose It Sleep Review

- Why you sleep is a mystery to scientists. We do know it's a critical window for your immune system, hormonal health, and psychological health, specifically true of the hours between 11:00 p.m. and 4:00 a.m.
- If you cannot sleep, investigate your cortisol, blood sugar control, inflammation, melatonin-blocking activities (i.e., blue light exposure), and even progesterone levels for some women. Looking into your caffeine hygiene and getting investigated for sleep apnea may also be helpful.
- The hormones affected by sleep are numerous. With a lack of sleep, you can get stuck in a fat-storing mode and develop elevated blood glucose and insulin levels. It is also common to start to feel hungry all the time, to have your metabolism slow (leptin and ghrelin), and to experience a decrease in baseline activity levels or NEAT. Growth and repair, muscle development, and anti-aging effects are attributed to growth hormone, which is also released during sleep.
- Set a bedtime hour and routine. Avoid blue light and stimulating activities before bed.
- If lifestyle interventions fail, then low-dose melatonin, magnesium, and / or herbal formulas may be what you need to refine your sleep hygiene. If you find that these aren't enough, check in with a doctor to better understand the root cause (inflammation, infection, high cortisol, etc.) of your sleep issues.

TODAY I CREATE A

STRESS-FREE

WORLD FOR MYSELF.

—LOUISE HAY

4

THE TRUTH ABOUT STRESS AND YOUR WAISTLINE

Stress has an undeniable and significant effect on weight loss. Long-term stress increases your appetite and cravings. It will jack up your inflammation levels and change the hormones associated with fat loss. In the face of stress, perceived or physiological, you can be exhausted, feel as if you are aging at a rapid rate, and get stuck in fat storage mode. Stress isn't always as obvious as you might think. There are many hidden sources of stress that must be uncovered in order for you to break out of the weight loss resistance cycle.

Stress is simply your body's hormonal response to your environment, which differs depending on what is going on around you. There is an acute stress response, defined by the hormone adrenaline (epinephrine), and a chronic stress response, defined by changes in cortisol patterns. They each have very different effects on your weight loss. Stressors, those widely varied factors that bring about a stress response, seem to be pervasive. In the age of social media, we live in a state of constant comparison and never-ending connectedness, a state of overwork, and innovation moves faster than we could ever hope to keep up with. Many of you will identify as frazzled, stressed out, overwhelmed perfectionists or over achievers. And these are just the visible and perceived stressors! It is not only what you see that can be contributing to your weight loss resistance. Did you know that hidden infections, blood sugar imbalances, food intolerances, nutrient deficiencies, and bacterial imbalances in our gut are also chronic stressors? These physiological stressors may also be stealing your health, energy, and vitality.

Let's jump into a primer on the nervous system, because there are different types of stress—and they are not all bad.

The Autonomic Nervous System

You have two arms of your autonomic nervous system, i.e., the nervous system that controls the function of your internal organs. One is known as the parasympathetic response, when we rest and digest. This is also when the hormone reset, relaxation, and repair modes of your body occur. The other arm is the sympathetic system, also known as fight or flight response. In this mode your body prioritizes survival, not relatively "non-essential" functions such as digestion or the immune response. This fight or flight mode is what we consider the classic stress response.

The Autonomic System

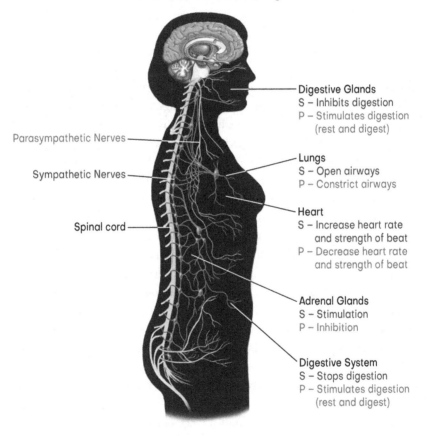

Parasympathetic Nerves

Sympathetic Nerves

Spinal cord

Digestive Glands
S – Inhibits digestion
P – Stimulates digestion
(rest and digest)

Lungs
S – Open airways
P – Constrict airways

Heart
S – Increase heart rate
and strength of beat
P – Decrease heart rate
and strength of beat

Adrenal Glands
S – Stimulation
P – Inhibition

Digestive System
S – Stops digestion
P – Stimulates digestion
(rest and digest)

Figure 6. The autonomic nervous system's two branches, the parasympathetic (P) (the rest and digest system) and the sympathetic (S) (the fight or flight system), work opposite each other, affecting nearly every organ function in the body.

Table 2. Summary of the autonomic nervous system functions

Sympathetic Nervous System (Fight or Flight)	Parasympathetic Nervous System (Rest and Digest)
• Prepares the body to escape from stressful situations • Increases the heart rate and blood pressure • Pupils dilate to see better • Sweating starts and hairs stand up • Blood and energy diverted from digestion and certain areas of the brain.	• Supports proper moment to moment organ function • Slows the heart rate and decreases blood pressure • Eyes become less sensitive to light and stimulation • Sweating only as appropriate for temperature control • Digestion occurs and clear thinking with appropriate responses

Acute Stress

Picture this: After a long day at work you and your best friend decided to go to a bar near her house. When you got there, there was no parking, so you park on a dark side street. When it's time to leave the bar, after one too many drinks and two too many hours, you and your friend part ways, and you begin to walk to your car. You notice that a man, who left the bar behind you, is still following you as you enter a less populated and darker street. At this point you are nervous, your mind starts to race, your heart is pumping, muscles are tensing, your hair is standing up on end, and you begin to hear every sound, smell every scent. Your pupils start to dilate, searching for light, and your peripheral vision widens. You quicken your pace and anxiety is getting the best of you. You are primed to run at any second.

The acute stress response is primitive. Your body responds to acute stressors with the same life or death intensity that it would have had ten thousand years ago, when people were chased by predators. You are primed to feel everything, see everything, and to escape a perceived threat. Today, although our acute stressors have changed, our bodies respond the same way to such things as perfectionism, an unexpected email, traffic jams, and being late to a meeting.

So, what happens internally when acute stress strikes? First, the stress signals are perceived in your brain by an area known as the hypothalamus. From here the sympathetic nervous system (fight or flight) kicks into action, stimulating a release of norepinephrine and epinephrine from the adrenal medulla and your nerve endings. This acute stress response readies your body for quick action, increasing your heart rate and directing blood flow to your heart and muscles so you can run from that bear! Blood is directed away from other organs, such as your digestive tract and certain areas of your brain. When an organ doesn't get proper blood flow, it's not able to function properly. (And we wonder why we are bloated and foggy-headed all day!)

The other functions of norepinephrine and epinephrine include increasing the amount of blood glucose available to your muscles so that you have the fuel to escape, should you need it, or not. These hormones are necessary signals for body fat breakdown, known as counter regulatory hormones. Keep them in mind as we move forward.

By now, you may be thinking, I'm not a perfectionist, my life is pretty cushy, and I don't frequent dark alleys. But if you think that means you're not stressed, I have news for you. First of all, the acute stress response, those seconds after a perceived stressor, don't actually have a detrimental effect on the metabolism. In fact, epinephrine and norepinephrine can help you to burn fat. It's only when we have *constant* perceived stressors (emails at work, traffic jams, and relationship stress) or the effects of the internal physiological stressors (inflammation, infection, blood sugar issues, diet), which we are about to dive into, that we get the chronic stress response. This is where the problematic issues truly lay.

The Stress Response

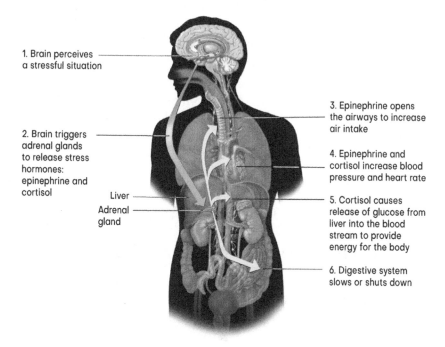

1. Brain perceives a stressful situation

2. Brain triggers adrenal glands to release stress hormones: epinephrine and cortisol

Liver

Adrenal gland

3. Epinephrine opens the airways to increase air intake

4. Epinephrine and cortisol increase blood pressure and heart rate

5. Cortisol causes release of glucose from liver into the blood stream to provide energy for the body

6. Digestive system slows or shuts down

Figure 7: When you perceive a stressful event, the body's stress response kicks into action. With a chronic stress activation, digestion decreases, adrenals are forced to work overtime, and glucose levels rise. The downstream effects of this response are an increased insulin demand, lowering glucose, and long-term fat storage.

Chronic Stress

When we talk about chronic stress it rarely involves one stressor. What it *does* involve is cortisol, a stress hormone, which also comes from the adrenal cortex. Cortisol is involved in almost every aspect of our health. After cortisol is released from the adrenal gland, it is circulated in the bloodstream, where it reaches our different organs and tissues. There are receptors for cortisol on almost every tissue in the body, meaning that it can change the function of each organ individually. Although it has many important roles in the body, we don't want it too high or too low, or high or low at the wrong times (see fig. 8 below). Ideally, cortisol release should be on a circadian rhythm: high in the morning, waking you up, and then a slow decline throughout the day to its lowest point at night. (This allows melatonin to rise so that you can go to sleep.)

The Circadian Rhythm of Cortisol with Chronic Stress

Cortisol and Circadian Rhythm

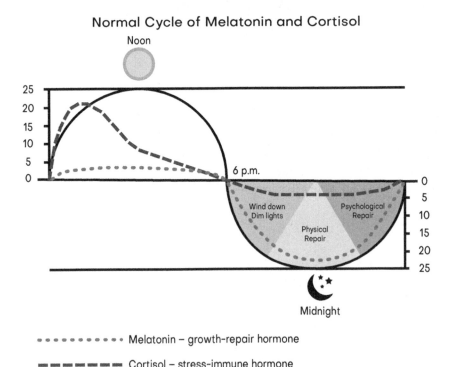

Normal Cycle of Melatonin and Cortisol

•••••••••••• Melatonin – growth-repair hormone

━━ ━━ ━━ ━━ Cortisol – stress-immune hormone

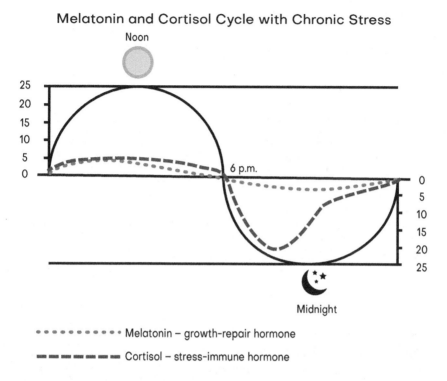

Figure 8: Cortisol is meant to be released on a circadian rhythm, rising first thing in the morning, spiking as soon as you open your eyes, and then dropping steadily throughout the day, allowing for melatonin to increase and sleep to begin at night. If cortisol rhythms are altered then sleep and melatonin synthesis are disrupted and physical and psychological repair benefits are lost.

Here's the kicker: when cortisol patterns are off, you can have a whole host of symptoms.

- Anxiety or depression
- Fatigue
- Brain fog
- Inflammation
- Immune system issues or autoimmune conditions
- Poor sleep (either a struggle to fall to sleep or waking up, specifically between 2:00 a. m. and 4:00 a.m.)
- Sugar, salt, and fat cravings
- Hormonal imbalances (losing your period, heavy period, intense cramps, PMS, infertility)

- Bloating, ulcers, and digestive issues
- Weight gain (specifically in the belly and upper back)
- Metabolic syndrome (diabetes, high cholesterol, and high blood pressure)

This list doesn't even cover the entire gamut, but I think you get the picture.

Table 3: Summary of the acute stress versus chronic stress response

Acute Stress Response	Chronic Stress Response
Predominantly epinephrine and norepinephrine	Predominantly cortisol
<ul><li>Increased heart rate</li><li>Increased blood pressure</li><li>Sugar stores (glycogen) converted to glucose by liver</li><li>Lungs opened for more breathing</li><li>Blood diverted from digestive system and brain</li><li>Increased metabolism</li></ul>	<ul><li>Water retained</li><li>Glycogen and protein used for energy, increased blood glucose</li><li>Immune system suppressed or poorly regulated, autoimmune conditions</li><li>Healing inhibited</li></ul>

Take my patient Lee, for example. Lee commuted one hour both ways in traffic. She had a high-pressure job that she loved but the deadlines were taking their toll. Lee ate most of her meals in meetings, where she had little control over the egg and dairy content of those foods—two of her food sensitivities—or when she had a moment between meetings. This meant she was eating more carbohydrates than her body could handle; therefore, her blood sugar was on a rollercoaster. She was bloated and either felt wired or totally exhausted; there was no happy medium for her. No matter how much Lee exercised, or how few calories she ate, she could not lose the weight she wanted to from her midsection. This is the quintessential presentation of chronic stress and an altered cortisol response.

The Physiology behind the Chronic Stress Response

As mentioned, cortisol is the main hormone that inflicts chaos on the body in the chronic stress response. We've reviewed the symptoms you can experience when you have an altered cortisol rhythm, but how exactly does cortisol make you feel frumpy, frustrated, hangry, and inflamed? Let's take a look.

- It regulates blood glucose levels. When your blood sugar drops, or in an emergency, cortisol can grab glucose from your other tissues (liver, muscles) and then pump it into the bloodstream.

- It lowers leptin, a hormone that tells your body how many fat stores you have, in the short term. It also stops your brain from listening to leptin over the long term. This increases your hunger and your drive to food, lowers your metabolism, and makes you more tired.
- It regulates your immune system. Both an overactive and underactive immune system are related to altered cortisol patterns. You need cortisol to keep your inflammation levels in check.
- It regulates water control at the level of the kidney and, therefore, your blood pressure, water retention, and frequency that you pee.
- It affects your skin integrity and healing.
- It affects your memory, mental clarity, and ability to recall information. (FYI, chronic stress can actually shrink your hippocampus, a part of your brain involved in memory, learning, and emotion!)

"YOUR BODY IS SAYING, 'OH, NO, GIRLFRIEND, I HAVE YOUR BEST INTEREST IN MIND, SO I'M GOING TO DO EVERYTHING I CAN TO KEEP YOU LIVING FOR YEARS, WHICH MEANS WE HOLD ON TO YOUR FUEL STORES!'"

The Hormones behind Stress-Induced Weight Loss Resistance

At a basic level, hormones are the body's communication system. When you look at it this way, it makes sense that stress starts a cascade of communication about the safety of a body. If you were seeing friends getting let go at work and people were warning the layoffs were going to hit your department, you wouldn't empty your savings account on a new car, would you? Similarly, your body isn't going to "spend" its fat stores when it is getting messages that it may need those stores during upcoming hard times. The quintessential paradigm of weight loss resistance: your body is saying, "Oh, no, girlfriend, I have your best interest in mind, so I'm going to do everything I can to keep you living for years, which means we hold on to your fat stores!" Let's break down these hormonal influences.

Glucose and Insulin Galore

With stress and cortisol, the situation appears to be a double whammy for sticking you in fat storage mode. Not only does stress increase your blood glucose, which increases your insulin, but cortisol also increases your insulin resistance. It does this by releasing free fatty acids.[26-28] These free fatty acids change the way insulin can interact with the receptors. It's like someone puts gum in your lock: when you put the key in, the door won't open! This is insulin resistance, which as you will come to find in **chapter 6**, can trap you in fat-storing mode.[26,29] I will say this again: your body is smart. Every time you become stressed it gets primed to store more fat, to protect you from starving in the face of tomorrow's stress. Of course, the body doesn't realize that we are not actually experiencing a food shortage.

Since insulin gets its own chapter, we'll focus more here on glucose. We have all heard about the effects of elevated blood glucose on health. It's called diabetes. Diabetes increases your risk of kidney disease, contributes to poor healing, neurological changes, memory issues, cardiovascular disease, and so forth. Not the quality of life that myself or any of my patients are going for, that is for sure!

Even if your glucose isn't high all the time, blood sugar swings are a huge stress on the body. This puts you at increased risk of diabetes, heart disease, obesity, and Alzheimer's in the long term.

Sex Hormone Havoc

I know I said that we weren't going to discuss hormonal imbalances, but I have to mention them here because cortisol has such a profound effect on your sex and metabolic hormones.

Sex Hormone Balance

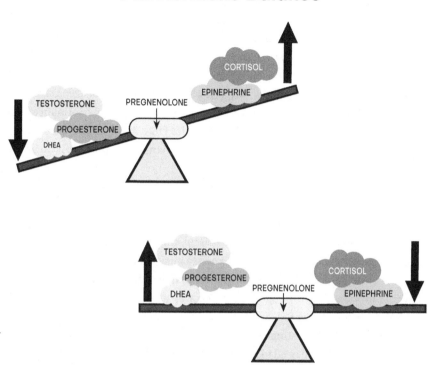

Figure 9: Stress has a huge impact on the hormonal balance of the body. An increase in cortisol and epinephrine (A) can function to decrease fat loss supportive hormones such as testosterone, progesterone, and DHEA. In an ideal state (B) we want to see cortisol and epinephrine in balance with your other hormones

One of the systems that I talk about all the time in my patient practice is the notion of adrenal hormone balance, which is commonly discussed as the *pregnenolone steal*. The concept is that the body's systems revolve around an axis of balance. All of our hormones function on a teeter-totter system, or feedback system, meaning that when one is elevated, the other decreases or vice versa. The actual feedback mechanism that occurs to change your female hormones in the face of stress is complex. The intricate details of this system is not what is important here, but the outcome on your weight loss resistance is! When in chronic stress, our adrenal glands will increase cortisol, and we often see lower adrenal progesterone production. This low progesterone is an epidemic of our generation. Progesterone (*pro-gestation*, meaning ability to carry a baby to term) comes from the adrenal glands and the ovaries and is important for fertility, having a sense of calm and for deep sleep as discussed in **chapter 3**. Progesterone is not the only hormone affected though. We also see other "male sex hormones" affected. These include the adrenal androgens DHEAs and testosterone.

We want just enough of DHEAs and testosterone, which at the right levels have been shown to protect against weight gain and support weight loss. Some studies have even shown that the ratio of DHEAs to cortisol is predictive of weight loss success in those having weight loss surgeries.[30] These adrenal androgens, again in the proper amounts, are also involved in our energy, exercise performance, the get-up-and-go feeling as I call it, and our libido. How many of you chronically stressed women are struggling with a low libido? Many, if my practice is an accurate representation.

Growth Hormone

As mentioned in **chapter 3**, growth hormone is yet another anabolic, weight loss supportive hormone that's critical to have circulating in appropriate amounts. The benefits of growth hormone have not seemed to breach mainstream media yet, but "hacking growth hormone" is something the bodybuilding community has been exploring for decades. Although I am in no way promoting taking growth hormone, there is something to learn here. When you do not have appropriate levels of growth hormone circulating, you can have poor exercise recovery. You just don't build the muscle that you need to increase your metabolism. Growth hormone also has anti-insulin benefits. Just as its name suggests, this hormone promotes growth and development, not fat storage. Cortisol and growth hormone seem to oppose each other, with cortisol breaking down muscle and increasing insulin. More cortisol, less growth hormone, less muscle building, less proper fuel usage, anti-aging and fat burning.

Stress and the Thyroid

The thyroid is the canary in the coal mine, and as we start to see a stress epidemic so, too, do we see a hypothyroid (or underactive thyroid) epidemic. This is not a coincidence. When you are stressed, one of the ways your body goes into protection mode is by downregulating your metabolism, i.e., slowing the number of calories your body burns throughout the day. There can be a decreased communication from your brain to your thyroid, with your brain saying, "Hold your horses, we just can't afford this kind of energy output right now." Issues in other parts of the body, such as the gut or liver, can also decrease the conversion of your storage thyroid hormone (T4) into your active hormone (T3). Finally, your thyroid can slam on the brakes through an increase in something called Reverse T3 (RT3), literally rearranging the shape of the active hormone so that it's not active anymore and slows down the metabolism further. Thyroid hormones have umpteen functions in the body, so this effect can lead to everything from even further imbalanced sex hormones to fatigue, constipation, poor detoxification, depression, dry skin, aches and pains, and weight gain.

In short, if cortisol is activated chronically, then your hormones are bound to be messed up. The work here is not to correct the hormones themselves but to correct the cause of the imbalance. You wouldn't continue to bail out a boat if you could see the leak. You would focus your attention on plugging the hole, shutting down the source of the issue, and only then would you focus on getting your bailing buckets to empty out the boat. The same mindset applies here, and we'll explore it in the strategies below.

Leptin

The final hormone signalling system to consider is how cortisol affects leptin, which controls appetite and satiety. Cortisol functions to lower leptin in the short term, increasing our hunger and drive to food, and lowering our basal metabolic rate and drive toward movement. On the other hand, chronic cortisol also affects the proper regulation of our immune system and can leave us in a state of chronic low-grade inflammation. This inflammation can contribute to leptin resistance, meaning your brain doesn't hear the signal from your fat cells so it thinks that your body is lean.

Do you ever feel like you could eat everything in sight and still not be full? Do you feel like you have to use your willpower throughout the day to prevent yourself from constantly snacking or indulging in those comfort foods? Do you feel like your metabolism just keeps slowing down, or is broken altogether? You may have to drag your butt to the gym and find that your innate drive is much more toward the couch than the park. You are not alone if this is where you find yourself now. Although a few different factors contribute to leptin resistance, stress is a major player.

"IT IS SOCIALLY ACCEPTABLE TO HAVE A LINE OF COOKIES AT A PARTY FOR PEOPLE TO ENJOY, BUT MOST OF US WOULD NOT SERVE UP LINES OF COCAINE."

Why Do We Crave Comfort Foods?

Did you know your body rewards you for eating after a stressful period? Studies have been done showing that Oreos interact with the brain in a way that is almost identical to cocaine![31] Can you imagine? It is socially acceptable to have a line of cookies at a party for people to enjoy, but most of us would not serve up lines of cocaine. Yet, the sugary processed food does the same thing to our brains: a similar reward, a similar high, a similar escape from reality, and a similar dose of pleasure. And then we wonder why the only thing that we can think about at 3:00 p.m. is the cake on the table at the office. Well, here's your answer: you are craving a dopamine hit!

When you eat hyper-palatable foods (high sugar, high fat, and high carbs), your body will downregulate the stress response. No wonder comfort foods are labelled as such; they can physiologically comfort your brain and lower the stress response.[32]

You might have guessed that cortisol has a role to play in all this: it works in our brain to increase the reward we feel when we do eat. This is one of the other evolutionary "protective mechanisms" you may have heard about. When you are stressed your body wants you to eat, and it wants you to store that food! That is how it protects you from dying in a famine, or ensures that you have fuel to run from that bear. So not only do we crave comfort foods (the beloved chocolate cake, mac and cheese, pizza, and spaghetti), but any foods. My philosophy is when you know, you grow, meaning you can be empowered to work with your body in states of stress and overwhelm.

The information that I've shared above is just the tip of the iceberg when it comes to understanding how chronic stress affects your metabolism and fat loss potential. I keep my pulse on this research, and researchers are constantly learning of new ways that your system gets sabotaged by stress. The takeaway here is check in with your stress. To help you do that, choose which of the main stressors below is your primary one.

"I SEE SOME PEOPLE WHO CAN (OMPLETELY ELIMINATE THEIR STRESS, EXHAUSTION, ANXIETY, SENSE OF OVERWHELM, ANGER, DEPRESSION, AND BRAIN FOG SIMPLY BY BALANCING THEIR BLOOD SUGAR."

Perceived Chronic Stressors

Stress Addiction and a Need for External Approval

Stress addiction is a real issue in modern society. We seem to equate "busy" with "important." Many people use "insanely busy" to describe their days as if it gives them street cred. So why do we glorify busy, and why do so many of us struggle to slow down, relax, and say no to projects? Well it starts in the brain of course!

When you engage in an activity that causes stress, your initial response is the production of epinephrine, norepinephrine, and your natural opiates, known as *beta endorphins*. Both the adrenaline rush and the endorphin rush (commonly known as the runner's high) can stimulate good feelings. Some Type A go-getters can become addicted to these feel-good chemicals, perpetually looking for their next hit. Without even knowing it, some of you derive a hedonistic kind of pleasure from putting yourselves into stressful situations. Have you ever procrastinated on a project, knowing that you were going to have to hustle against a deadline to get it done? Do you often take on more projects than you should, knowing it will overwhelm you? Do you find yourself justifying stressful behaviours or staying in a high-paced environment that you know is making you sick, all while knowing you have other options? Do you consistently miss out on time with family and friends because of projects you have taken on? If this is you, then you may be caught in a cycle of addiction.

If you identify yourself in this category then getting out of this cycle might be particularly hard for you. Relaxation and prioritizing yourself sound good, but it's likely that you have tried these things before. As we go through these next sections, it will be critical for you to eliminate as many of the other physiological issues as possible, and you will also be a great candidate for adaptogenic herbs. These herbs help to support your stress levels and mental health while you are overcoming physiological addiction or burnout. (More on these soon.) You will need to schedule self-care and endorphin-boosting activities, and you will need accountability. The partner you have selected to come on this journey with you can be a great person to support you. Keep this in mind and make sure to schedule your health into your priority list!

Physiological, or Internal, Stressors

Blood Sugar Dysregulation

Blood sugar swings are the silent stress epidemic of the modern world. I see some people who can completely eliminate their stress, exhaustion, anxiety, sense of overwhelm, anger, depression, and brain fog simply by balancing their blood sugar. Did you know that eating carbohydrates, such as fruit, crackers, bread, or juice, on their own can cause a rapid rise and fall in your blood sugar? When you are not eating a well-balanced meal or snack (or are missing good-quality fat, protein, and fibre), your food quickly leaves the stomach and enters the intestines. This can cause a spike in your blood sugar that the digestive and other metabolic systems can't keep up with, kind of like a flash flood. Then, as your insulin levels are finally able to rise, digestive enzymes kicking into action, the elevated blood sugar plummets, swinging too low because of the overcompensation. Both high and low blood sugar have similar symptoms of shakiness, anxiety, feelings of overwhelm, fatigue, lack of concentration, moodiness, and—you guessed it—anger.

Your blood sugar is a very tightly controlled system because your brain requires glucose to properly function. Therefore, when your blood sugar drops too low, your body has to use cortisol to liberate glucose to raise your blood sugar. This system can then overshoot, causing too much glucose release, and the cycle starts again. So many of your body's resources can become dedicated to blood glucose regulation, a system that further messes with your fat-storing capacity, your appetite, and your goals to feel well and be in a body that reflects that.

Adya was the perfect example of the power of blood sugar dysregulation on vitality and weight. In Adya's culture, rice, flour, and beans were central to the diet. It was quiet common to have a bowl of rice as a snack, skipping any vegetable, protein, or fat. When she came to me, she carried all of her weight in her abdomen and back; her arms and legs were lean. Adya was totally exhausted throughout the day, she woke up tired, got easily overwhelmed, and we laughed that her superpower was sleep onset. Given the opportunity, she could sleep on the bus, on a plane, at her desk, even in a meeting once. In addition to not losing weight despite her increasingly difficult (and exhausting) workouts, Adya was getting more and more anxious.

It was obvious to me that Adya's blood sugar was out of control. All of those carbs she was ingesting were sending her on an exhausting rollercoaster throughout the day. It was also affecting her mood and causing fat to stick like glue to her waistline. We had to shift the amount of carbohydrates Adya was eating and increase her protein, fat, fibre, and minimize her snacking. I was strict with Adya because I knew her potential to feel better and lose weight.

Adya, desperate to feel like she was contributing to the world again and to understand why her body felt like it was working against her, followed my directions to a T. She changed her diet completely, and within days she felt her energy increase, her productivity improve, and with the addition of adaptogens (there's a selection listed below), she stopped needing naps. These were the first signs of success. In Adya's case, her "waist loss," as we decided to call it, came quite quickly as well. She lost one full dress size within six weeks and continued to lose another one month after that.

> "WHEN [CERTAIN] NUTRIENTS ARE DEPLETED IN YOUR BODY, IT'S LIKE YOU ARE MISSING A WHEEL ON YOUR CAR. YOU SIMPLY CANNOT FUNCTION PROPERLY, AND IT'S INCREDIBLY STRESSFUL TO GET ANYWHERE."

Nutrient Deficiencies

There is no doubt that we are a culture that is overfed and undernourished. When you look at any packaged foods, it's blatantly obvious. They are filled with sugar, carbohydrates, poor-quality fats, and inflammatory, cheap proteins. Even our vegetables and fruits are depleted of minerals due to many of the current farming practices. It can be incredibly difficult to get all that we need from our foods these days.

Many of my patients ask me how it's possible for nutrient deficiencies to cause a stress response in the body. The answer is, of course, complicated. One recent study exploring nutrient depletions in the USA demonstrated that the most common nutrient deficiencies include iron, vitamin D, vitamin B6, vitamin A, vitamin E, vitamin C, folate, magnesium, and choline.[33] These nutrients are critical to many of the energy production, cell turnover, detoxification, immune system, and hormonal regulation systems of the body. When these nutrients are depleted in your body, it's like you are missing a wheel on your car. You simply cannot function properly, and it's incredibly stressful to get anywhere. Although it can be challenging to get these nutrients from our foods, the meal plans provided in **chapter 9** outline the best foods to eat to help keep you nourished. Some of you will likely require supplementation of specific nutrients as well. For women, these often include magnesium, vitamin D, iron, and folate (if you are of reproductive age). We'll return to subject of nutrients that have the most research for overcoming weight loss resistance, but first, we need to look at other hidden stressors.

Food Intolerances

Food intolerance and food allergies are very different things. You may not have an anaphylactic response (meaning you get hives, struggle to breathe, and your throat closes) to gluten or dairy, but many of you will simply not feel good when you eat them. This is an example of an intolerance. Food intolerances can increase the inflammation in your gut, which can then circulate throughout your body. In a healthy system, the body should recognize that small proteins are food and are therefore friend, not foe. In the case of food intolerances, a large protein interacts with the immune system in the digestive tract, and a certain arm of your immune system increases, known as the *IgG immune response*. This activation is a stress on your body.

As discussed, cortisol levels affect the way that your body deals with inflammation; it is an *immunosuppressant*. Therefore, cortisol can also help to lower the inflammation and decrease its impact on your health. (If you have ever been on prednisone, which is very similar to cortisol, then you know the anti-inflammatory nature.) Continually eating foods that you are sensitive to will trigger your internal system to try to minimize the impacts of inflammation and will therefore call on your stress hormones.

"IF YOU EXPERIENCE CHRONIC BLOATING, ABDOMINAL PAIN, CONSTIPATION, DIARRHEA, OR A COMBINATION OF ALL OF THESE, THEN YOU NEED TO CONSIDER IT AS A SIGN OF BODILY STRESS."

Gut Issues

Having had such horrible issues with my digestion for so many years, and having to protect my gut so fiercely, the effects of gut bacterial imbalances, *gut dysbiosis*, and leaky gut, *intestinal hyperpermeability*, are near and dear to my heart, and my stress response.

Not only do "bad bacteria" upregulate your immune system, causing low-grade inflammation, but they also increase the amount of food sensitivities you have and affect how well you absorb minerals and nutrients. If you experience chronic bloating, abdominal pain, constipation, diarrhea, or a combination of all of these, then you need to consider it as a sign of bodily stress. In fact the underlying cause of these symptoms can be a cause and a consequence of the stress response. These things can take their toll emotionally, but also can have a significant impact on your weight loss potential.

Infections

If you have an underlying viral or bacterial infection, such as Epstein-Barr virus, Lyme disease, H. pylori, streptococcal infections, sexually transmitted infections (STIs), or urinary tract infections (UTIs), that needs to be dealt with before you will be able to feel your best. Infections are a huge stress to the body. These are inflammatory by definition and they require a lot of resources to control. Imagine how you feel when you get a bad flu. Your body is definitely in protection mode. When you are sick, your body's goals are not to lose weight, increase your energy, and bounce you through the day with a positive outlook on life. The body's goal is to fight the infection and prevent death (because back in the days before medications, some of these infections were life-threatening). If you are experiencing chronic fatigue, joint aches, autoimmune conditions, thyroid conditions, or any other chronic disease state, then looking into this stress source may be important to get you on track to kicking your stress and meeting your weight loss goals. Working with a medical doctor or naturopathic doctor to rule these out is important to *every* aspect of your health.

Score Your Stress

The way any of these stressors manifest in your body is going to be very individual, depending on how long they have affected you and how many you experience—yes, it's possible to be afflicted with more than one of these hidden stressors. That's why I have developed the stress type quiz for you. The type of symptoms you experience will tell you more about the best treatment for you. Check the boxes below for the symptoms you experience.

Do you tend to … ?	Yes	No
Section A		
worry about big and small things		
be unable to stop worrying even when you try		
have pent up energy and could explode at any time		
have muscle spasms		
be sensitive to noise, smells, small movements		
find other people describe you as jumpy		
get hyper in response to events and can be up all night before a big meeting or speech		
be prone to diarrhea and stomach pain, even appetite changes		
sweat a lot		
have high blood pressure		
have a lot of nervous energy throughout the day and restlessness		
be highly emotional in general, whether laughing, crying, or easily angered		
Section B		
be tired throughout the day but at night your mind starts to race and you can't fall asleep easily		
have IBS with constipation and diarrhea		
find morning a difficult time of day with low energy and low appetite		
appear to be highly driven and motivated externally but internally feel burnt out and overwhelmed		
have salt and sweet cravings		
alternate between symptoms in Section A and Section C, depending on the day		

Do you tend to … ?	Yes	No
Section C		
experience exhaustion throughout the day, fall asleep easily, and wake feeling unrefreshed, no matter how many hours slept		
have muscle and joint pains and poorly healing wounds		
have poor exercise tolerance and recovery (can feel weak and achy during and after)		
have low blood pressure		
frequently get sick with colds and flus		
crave salts and sweets		
have dark circles under your eyes		
have constipation and/or reflux and indigestion		
have a tendency toward low mood and apathy		
get dizzy or light-headed when standing from lying or sitting		
lack motivation and energy to focus and stay on task		

Mostly A's—On Alert

You are in adrenal overdrive, your body responding to life as if it were an acute stress. It is going to be critical to reprogram your responses with mindfulness but also calming herbs. Cortisol and adrenaline are likely raging through your body day and night and are ready to throw you into action.

Mostly B's—Wired and Tired

In this situation your body cannot handle the constant stress throughout the day. You are coping but likely needing uppers in the morning (coffee) and downers at night (wine/alcohol). This is because you are making cortisol at the wrong time of day. Instead of getting your cortisol energy in the morning, yours is high at night, keeping you awake and anxious (see fig. 8). You are riding the line between On Alert and Burnout so fluctuations are common. It's time to get things in check before burnout hits.

Mostly C's—Burnout

Welcome to burnout. I am sure that you did not need to take that quiz to understand that your body is overwhelmed and shutting down. You need to work on reducing your stress levels, and building yourself back up is also going to be a critical component. Your cortisol, your get-up-and-go, stays in bed and isn't in the mood to see the light of day. This has significant impact on your health, vitality, and weight.

Grab your workbook at **www.sarahwilsonnd.com/loseitbookbonus** and list your top five stressors in the stress inventory section. Here you will also record your starting score for the quiz above to be able to compare once you read below about how to prioritize your stress-busting activities. Remember, with all of the quizzes in this book it's important to repeat them after embarking on the program. This helps you to see how far you have come, but also to see what work still needs to be done.

Stress Busters

Although stress seems ubiquitous in today's society, there are so many things that can be done to minimize its effects. We will never live completely stress-free lives ladies and that's in no way my goal for you because it isn't realistic. Instead, see where you can shift your activities, shift your perspective, to meet your goals *all* while living your life. As I said, we have a stress epidemic, but only you can take that first step toward feeling amazing and living up to your full potential!

Walking in Nature

Walking in nature is one of my favourite activities to cut the stress and get back into my body. It is almost like a walking meditation. Studies have shown that walking lowers your cortisol and the nature aspect is also critical. There is a process known as forest bathing, or Shinrin-yoku, that has been studied in Japan for decades. Researchers have found that forest bathing activities help to regulate cortisol, lower blood pressure and heart rate, improve the immune system, and improve the sense of well-being and energy.[34,35] Whether it's the oxygen, the essential oils in the air, or the process of disconnecting from the rush of the city, I do not know. What I *do* know is that it works like a charm for me and nearly every patient I have recommended this to. It is the foundation of a stress-reduction, fat loss plan.

"THE MORAL OF THE STORY IS THAT CUDDLING MORE, HAVING MORE SEX, AND BEING AROUND PEOPLE YOU LOVE IS GREAT FOR YOUR STRESS RESPONSE, AND YOUR WAISTLINE!"

Oxytocin and Your Waistline

When was the last time that you felt deeply in love? The kind of love that warms your heart and settles your mind. Think about that feeling for a second; I bet you can just feel your stress response calming. That's because of every woman's best friend, oxytocin. Oxytocin and cortisol are antagonists, on opposite ends of the tee-ter-totter, so that when oxytocin is high, the effects of cortisol are low and vice versa.

Oxytocin, increased in the body by cuddling, sex, laughter, social support, and breastfeeding, has been shown to offset the effects of stress in the body. I do not think we can underestimate this one. New studies are suggesting that not only does oxytocin increase resilience to stress, specifically in post-traumatic stress disorder, but that it also may be useful in managing diabetes and reducing obesity.[36,37] The moral of the story is that cuddling more, having more sex, and being around people you love is great for your stress response, and your waistline! Win-win!

Yoga and Mindfulness

Over-exercise is as detrimental as under-exercise for the metabolism. Often the switch from abusive pounding workouts to challenging but nourishing yoga work-outs can make all the difference. That is why yoga and breathing exercises are non-negotiable with many women who have been pushing their bodies and still not losing weight. There is nothing quite like a thirty-day yoga experience to change your perception, stress levels, anxiety, and your body! Not to mention the mental/emotional stress-reduction benefits of yoga.

One patient specifically, Alice, found herself waking every day at 5:30 a.m. to get in an intense workout. She pushed herself hard six mornings a week, on top of an incredibly fast-paced life. She found herself gaining weight, having all sorts of digestive issues, and not recovering from her exercise the way she used to. She felt completely exasperated. Alice felt that she was "eating right" and working out, so why the weight gain? This is an incredibly common scenario. If you are sacrificing sleep, eating too few calories, eating the wrong foods at the wrong times, and stressing yourself out with workouts on top of a stressful life, then a slower metabolism and weight gain are a natural protection response for the body.

In Alice's case, I put her on an intense workout ban and overhauled her diet to ensure she ate the right carbohydrates at the right time, enough fat, and plenty of anti-inflammatory nutrient-dense foods. The only thing Alice could fit into her schedule was a regular yoga class and a breathing routine, so this was where we started. Yoga has been shown in the research to support proper cortisol production and can lower anxiety and depressive symptoms.[38] Yoga has also been shown to increase the antioxidant status of the body twofold, to lower inflammation, and to lower epinephrine (adrenaline).[39] On this plan, Alice had more energy and stopped getting injured during her workouts. She also eliminated a decade of constipation and bloating. Like Alice, you too can nourish yourself with a yoga and mindfulness practice and still drop from 32% to 26% body fat.

Take a Breath

Breathing is also under-emphasized. We have to do it anyway, so we might as well do it right. One simple exercise is known as box breathing, or controlled breathing in the literature. The goal here is to sit in a comfortable position, upright and stable. Then you breathe in through your nose for four seconds, hold your breath for four seconds, breathe out through your mouth for four seconds, hold and repeat. This exercise, repeated even five times can leave you feeling a whole world of different! Try it now.

Gratitude Journaling

I find that gratitude journaling and keeping an "attitude of gratitude" are critical to managing stress. Even changing the conversation here from *I have to* to *I get to* can make a huge difference to your outlook on life. And it's in fact your perception that is the key determinant to whether you become stressed or not.

Recall the scenario in which you imagined you were walking on a dark street. The perception of danger is what triggered the body's stress response in that example. Although that perception turned out to be false, we put ourselves in a similarly perceived stressful position all day long! How exhausting, right? Focusing on gratitude instead can alter your perception and, therefore, limit the metabolism-breaking chronic stress response. I have included my gratitude journal template in your workbook. (See **www.sarahwilsonnd.com/loseitbookbonus**.) The goal here is to think of at least three things you are grateful for, one to two times per day. (Bonus points if you share these things with your accountability partner.) I focus on the morning and right before bed. I also use I get to throughout the day to reframe my perceptions. This strategy is a game changer for so many women!

"WHEN YOU COME TO NOURISH YOURSELF, ACTING OUT OF SELF-LOVE INSTEAD OF SELF-ABUSE WILL CHANGE YOUR WORLD, YOUR PERSPECTIVE, YOUR CRAVINGS, AND YOUR BODY!"

Kick the Restrict Mentality

There's no doubt about it, ladies, we are in a culture that empowers and idolizes the restriction mentality. We cannot avoid discussions of fewer carbs, fewer calories, lower fat, and lower sugar. We see hashtags with no pain no gain, less is more, and we idolize celebrities who restrict themselves into a socially acceptable size. But let's also face facts: advantages such as a personal chef, a personal trainer, a schedule that sets you up for two hours of exercise daily, a massage therapist, and a personal assistant make a certain lifestyle easier to maintain. It is also easy to compare yourself, judge yourself, and resent the lack of progress that you have seen. I urge you to take these first steps I am proposing in this book to slowly and surely move toward a world of nourishment.

Research has shown over and over again that those who restrict themselves also have a tendency to binge or at the very least experience an elevated hunger level that makes the experience of day-to-day eating an exercise of willpower and mental anguish.[32,40] When you are struggling with weight loss resistance, it's common to feel as though food is the enemy and that your body is betraying you. I am here to guide you through the experience of recognizing and overcoming your obstacles, empowering you to reach your goals while loving, or at least appreciating, the body you are in. Kicking the restrictive mentality goes a long way toward achieving that attitude. When you come to nourish yourself, acting out of self-love instead of self-abuse will change your world, your perspective, your cravings, and your body!

Adaptogens

Medicinal herbs, what we call adaptogens, have been used for centuries and have historically caused wars because of their value to nations. I use adaptogens every day in my practice, with life-changing results. That said, I don't believe that you can supplement your way out of a crappy diet and lifestyle, so don't skip to this section without first exploring at least one of the options above.

Adaptogens work just as they sound, to help your body cope with the stress response and adapt to varying situations. The use of adaptogens is definitely where my East meets West medical brain comes into full force. I believe that where research studies exist, we need to consider them, but in some cases the traditional use across centuries truly stands for itself. Below are my favourite adaptogens for you to explore and try. You will notice that I've outlined them according to their best use as well as their individual properties. I encourage you to try some of them; if one isn't working for you in the first two weeks, then another may be better. Recall your stress type quiz results; the herbs listed in that specific category offer a starting place. For example, if your score categorized you as On Alert then read through the Relora, lavender, chamomile, and tulsi category to see which herb, or herbs, you want to try first.

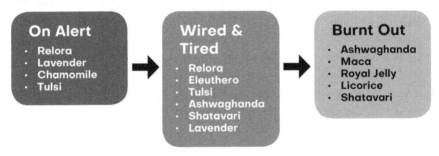

Adaptogens and Their Functions
Note: If you are on any prescription medications, are pregnant or trying to get pregnant, please check with your prescribing doctor before beginning any herbal supplements.

Ashwagandha (Withania somnifera)

Use and caution: A very versatile adaptogen in that it can help to regulate cortisol production, calm the mind in anxiety, and also produce a boost in energy. Ashwagandha has also been shown to improve thyroid function and is anti-inflammatory in nature.[41] As a bonus, traditionally Ashwagandha is used for both male and female libido and may have benefits to fertility. It belongs to the nightshade family, so it's best to avoid if sensitive to nightshades.

Dosage and time: Dried herb in a capsule 400–500 mg twice per day, morning and mid-afternoon. Tincture 50–60 drops twice per day in a small amount of water, in the morning and mid-afternoon.

Eleutherococcus senticosus

Use: My go-to herb in the case of mental exhaustion, need for physical performance, and also for night-shift workers and those with "social jetlag." Eleuthero can increase performance and decrease the perception of burnout.[42] This may be due to its ability to modulate neurotransmitters, chemical messengers in the brain. Eleuthero has been known as the revitalizer and is therefore in the more stimulating category of herbs. Despite this though it can help with recovery from burnout, unlike coffee, and improves the immune system.

Dosage and time: Dried herb in a capsule 500 mg twice per day in the morning and mid-afternoon. Tincture 60–100 drops three times per day in a small amount of water.

Holy Basil

Use: Also known as tulsi in the Ayurvedic tradition, where it's most commonly used to promote health and longevity, holy basil is a nourishing, stimulating herb that can protect the neurological system and increase energy. It may also decrease inflammation in the gut, which is critically important to reduce the triggers of the stress response to begin with. As a side benefit, tulsi may also help to regulate blood sugar and decrease the glucose and lipid response to a meal.

Dosage and time: Tea 1 tsp. of dried leaf in 8 oz. of water. Steep for 10 minutes covered and drink three times per day. Tincture 40–60 drops three times per day in a small amount of water.

Relora®

Use: This patented herbal formulation of Magnolia officinalis and Phellodendron amurense works wonders to calm the mind and decrease anxiety. Relora® has been shown to lower cortisol levels in stressed out women and can increase DHEAs, improve energy, and overall well-being.[43] As an added benefit, some studies show that Relora® can increase weight loss and decrease stress related eating.[44]

Dosage and time: Dried herbs in a capsule 250 mg twice per day, in the morning and evening.

Lavender

Use: This very calming herb can help with anxiety and racing thoughts. Lavender can be used as an inhaled essential oil, on your pillow, or can be consumed as a tea. Lavender likely is not directly changing cortisol levels, but it can symptomatically support mood.

Studies have shown that internal use of high-quality lavender essential oils (available in a pill form) can also be supportive of both anxiety and depression in a manner comparable to pharmaceuticals.[45] If exploring internal essential oil use, be sure to seek a healthcare provider because if the oil is improperly prepared or dosed it can be toxic.

Dosage and time: Tea 1 tsp. of dried flower in 8 oz. of water. Steep for 10 minutes covered, and drink twice per day. Essential oils can be used externally on pillows or in an Epsom salts bath to help to calm the body.

Chamomile

Use: The wonderful calming properties of this adaptogen decrease the stress response and help to calm anxiety. In addition, chamomile helps decrease digestive symptoms such as gas and abdominal cramping. Chamomile may also help to reduce constipation and promote regular bowel movements.

Dosage and time: Tea 1 tsp. of dried flower in 8 oz. of water. Steep for 10 minutes covered and drink twice per day.

Maca

Use: This is such a nourishing adaptogen for women. It helps to modulate hormones, increasing androgens which are protective for all the sex hormones. Maca can increase mental performance, improve libido and fertility, and increase energy. To be safe, do not use this herb if you have a history of estrogen-sensitive cancers.

Dosage and time: Dried herb in a capsule 750–1000 mg per day. Whole powder 1 Tbsp. per day.

Royal Jelly

Use: This is what I call a non-classical adaptogen. It has been used in fertility for decades due to its ability to increase DHEAs and boost egg quality.[46,47] This can offer protective benefits to the stress response. Research has also suggested that royal jelly can decrease blood glucose levels and modulate inflammation.[47,48] Although this is not proven in the research, if you have an allergy to bees it may be best to avoid royal jelly, as that is the source of this substance.

Dosage and time: Dried powder in a capsule 1–3 g per day in two divided doses.

Shatavari

Use: Also known as Asparagus racemosus, which translates to "she who has hundreds of husbands" (that, in itself, sounds exhausting!). It is a beautiful tonic for women that can enhance physical strength, memory, youthfulness, and fertility. It works to support adrenal function and can also increase estrogen levels in some women. To be safe, do not use this herb if you have a history of estrogen-sensitive cancers.

Dosage and time: Tincture 40–80 drops, three times per day in a small amount of water.

Licorice

Use: Also known as Glycyrrhiza glabra, this herb is saved for cases of burnout in my office. Licorice works to increase energy and decrease perception of burnout because it increases the circulating cortisol in the body. Licorice is also immuno-modulating, has benefits to blood sugar, and can decrease the histamine response in the gastrointestinal tract. Not only does licorice increase cortisol, but it can also increase blood pressure. If you have high blood pressure or hypertension then it's best to avoid this herb.

Dosage and time: Dried herb in a capsule 200–300 mg twice per day.

Other Supplements

Although not an adaptogen, one of my other favourite stress-reduction supplements is phosphatidylserine (PS), which helps to lower cortisol in response to stress. It can be very supportive to those who are in the On Alert and Wired & Tired phases, where cortisol can be elevated.[49–51] This should not be used if you are in Burnt Out phase though, as lowering cortisol is exactly the opposite of what you should be doing!

I often start patients on 100 mg mid-afternoon and before bed to help lower their nighttime cortisol. This should not be taken in the morning unless you have fight or flight symptoms from the moment you wake up. Dosages up to 600 mg have been used in the research, but I rarely see dosages over 400 mg provide more benefit. Aim to go low and slow with increases, and if fatigue or mental fog begin to increase, then lower or stop PS altogether.

Take Action

I'm going to ask you to push your limits throughout this book, because, let's be honest, what you've tried up to now hasn't worked, or you wouldn't be reading this book. You owe it to yourself to try something new. There is always resistance whenever I ask someone to find time in their day for self-care or to start to work on reframing stress. We feel time-poor, but the first step is to map out your day and look for spaces for quiet, cuddling, and rejuvenating activities. We all have them when we get organized a take a closer look. In the workbook provided you will find a time map planner (see **www.sarahwilsonnd.com/loseitbookbonus**). Use this to map out when you have time, even if it's 10 minutes to go for a walk or do some relaxing yoga (not power yoga). Then schedule it in. Scheduling, although it may feel rigid in the beginning, can be a godsend to lowering stress, because structure is what allows for fluidity, space, and creativity.

Challenge your beliefs today about what is possible for you to incorporate, and then slowly you will find that the self-care, gratitude journaling, supplementation, and mental reframing come naturally. Start with possibility!

The Finally Lose It Stress Review

- Our neurological system is very primitive. In fact, we have the same fight or flight stress response sitting in traffic or fighting with our spouse as we do running from a life-threatening situation.
- There are two stress responses, acute and chronic.
- In the acute phase we see quick changes to norepinephrine and epinephrine, followed by cortisol, a delayed response. This will rise and fall, affecting fat storage positively, if anything, because these hormones allow the use of fat to make glucose, or energy, for activity. In the short term this is supportive to fat loss.
- In the chronic phase, when cortisol is chronically elevated, or dysregulated, it will increase glucose inappropriately, forcing insulin to take the glucose from your bloodstream and put it into fat cells, locking it there. Chronic stress can also lead to inflammation and insulin resistance, where more and more insulin comes in to deal with glucose and even further trap us in a sugar-burning state.
- Chronic stress affects reproductive hormones, growth and repair hormones, the thyroid, and your appetite and cravings. This can leave us exhausted, lacking a sex drive, struggling with fertility, and even premature aging.
- Stress is not just mental and emotional; physiological effects such as blood sugar swings, nutrient deficiencies, food intolerances, gut bacterial imbalance, and underlying infections and inflammation are also forms of stress.
- The first step in reversing the stress response is identifying it. Then activities such as walking in nature, yoga, breathing, cuddling, gratitude journaling, and mindset changes are key.
- Adaptogens can be helpful to support specific stress types. These are especially important when we are chronically stressed or perpetually burnt out and need support to build ourselves back up.

ALL **DISEASE** BEGINS IN THE **GUT.**

—HIPPOCRATES

5

IT'S CALLED BELLY FAT FOR A REASON

Digestive Hormones and Weight Loss Resistance

Although we often think about digestion in terms of eating and pooping, that is truly just an outward reflection of a process much more intricate. The *gut microbiota*—or the sum total of all the bacteria, yeast, and other organisms in our gastrointestinal system—involves a balance between good bugs and bad bugs. And that balance is critical to all aspects of our health, including weight loss. When it comes to weight loss resistance, most if not all women struggling experience an increase in inflammation and gut hormone imbalances. Both inflammation in the body and changes in gut hormones have a basis in changes in the gut microbiota. How that happens is what we'll explore next. The main hormones I discuss in this chapter are not female sex hormones but hormones that affect our sense of fullness (CCK, PYY, ghrelin, and GLP-1) and our insulin release and sensitivity (GIP, GLP-1). Research in this area is ever developing, but we are beginning to understand that more than half of our metabolic concerns may start in the gut. Turns out, it's called belly fat for a reason!

I remember the first time I heard "all disease begins in the gut." Part of me wanted to believe it, because my worst health always coincided with my worst digestive issues. But at the same time, if this dictum was so commonly accepted, I had to wonder why none of my doctors had talked to me about how imbalances in my gut could be causing my weight gain, hormonal imbalances, joint pain, and mental anguish. I was skeptical, but my digestive issues were so crippling that I had nothing to lose by testing the claim. At that point, nothing could be worse than my frustration, my dwindling confidence in my body's ability to be well, and my trips, in pain, in and out of the hospital. I began by eliminating certain foods to see how they might be affecting my health. Losing my joint pain, congestion, brain fog, and losing weight in one month really spurred my curiosity!

You may be thinking, well, I have tried eliminating foods and nothing happened, so this chapter must not be for me. Well, hold your horses, sister! Our dive into the gut is going far beyond food elimination. In fact, I often tell my patients we should not have to be doing these extensive food eliminations. Having done it myself, I know that taking away all of your sugar, dairy, gluten, corn, soy, etc., can be really hard! However, fixing your broken gastrointestinal system is going to be a critical piece of your puzzle if you suffer from any of the following symptoms, in addition to stubborn fat tissue:

- Joint pain
- Autoimmune conditions (rheumatoid arthritis, psoriasis, eczema, Hashimoto's, etc.)
- Brain fog
- Bloating and gas
- Constipation or diarrhea
- Nasal congestion or postnasal drip
- Allergies or persistent rashes
- Persistent infections
- Diabetes
- Cravings for sugar, sweets, carbs, etc.

 Jenna was a full-time manager, who had a part-time obsession with personal development. The girl seemingly had it all together. She worked out almost daily, but not too hard. She meditated and had the best self-care and mindset practice I had ever seen. She went to bed on time, woke up on time, got sunlight in the morning, and dimmed her lights at night. She ate when she was hungry and prioritized food quality. She was "doing all the right things," but she still weighed 30 lbs more than she wanted. When Jenna came to see me, she was grateful for the mindset and self-care practices she had, but she was quickly losing faith in her body and gaining frustration. She felt destined to be overweight the rest of her life and had no idea why. Like most of us, what I came to learn is that Jenna's path had not always been one of health.

Jenna was born via C-section and received a number of rounds of antibiotics as a child. She had struggled with her weight the majority of her life and had "tried every diet in history." Those restrictive diets had resulted in weight loss, but she would gain back the lost pounds, and maybe more, when she added back more diversity to her diet. Jenna also sought out a lot of personal development work because she had a history of stress and burnout. In her previous job, Jenna barely had time to eat and would throw down food in order to fuel her blood sugar swings. This carried into today, when she realized that she was barely tasting her food, rushing through meals and chewing only enough so that she could swallow. Jenna also had some seriously disruptive gut symptoms, such as bloating, gas, and even diarrhea at times, although she had never really tried to change that with medical treatment.

The current life Jenna was living was the best version she thought she could have. She had almost given up, but when her friend started seeing great results working with me, she decided to come see me as well.

Although we do not have adequate testing for some of the gut hormones at the moment, I had enough information about Jenna's case to believe that her yo-yo dieting and burnout had taken their toll on her gut hormones. To start with, the girl didn't chew! Instituting a 30-chew rule immediately changed her bloating and gas. Jenna's diet, which had taken her carbohydrate intake way too low to be sustainable and allowed for few polyphenols, was contributing to inflammation and bacterial imbalance.

 Polyphenols are phytochemicals, or plant protection mechanisms. They are naturally occurring food compounds that can act as antioxidants, protecting us against premature aging, heart disease, Alzheimer's disease, and, you guessed it, weight loss resistance. Foods rich in polyphenols are dark-coloured fruits and vegetables, tea, coffee, olive oil, spices, and wine.

When Jenna and I first started working together, she was unable to tolerate the fibre additions, so she opted for testing. We found systemic inflammation and insulin resistance, but also yeast and bacterial overgrowth. This result helped to explain why she wasn't doing well on her high-fat diet. Jenna was open to overhauling her diet and lifestyle, which is exactly what we did. She went on phase 2 of the diet plan (see **chapter 8**) and spent two months working to support her microbiome and gut hormones. During this period, Jenna's energy and mental clarity soared. Her skin became clearer, and she lost two pants sizes. Three months after making the changes, we were able to retest Jenna's insulin resistance and inflammation, both of which had improved significantly. Not only did she feel better, but Jenna also finally regained faith in her body—the end result that I want for each of you!

"WE KNOW THAT 60–80% OF OUR IMMUNE SYSTEM SITS IN OUR GUT. IT CONTROLS APPETITE, BLOOD SUGAR REGULATION, WHOLE BODY INFLAMMATION LEVELS, MOOD, AND BODY FAT LEVELS."

Digestion 101

We tend to think about our digestive tract as little more than a poop manufacturer. We take in food, it miraculously fuels us by allowing us to absorb nutrients, and then, somehow, if we are lucky, we will have one to three solid bowel movements a day, and carry on feeling light and flat-stomached into our next meal. What many people don't know is that our digestive system is not only a place for chewing, digesting, and absorbing foods, but it's also a control centre. The research in this area is ever evolving, but we now know that 60–80% of our immune system sits in our gut. It controls appetite, blood sugar regulation, whole body inflammation levels, mood, and body fat levels.

Here's what ideal, mechanical digestion looks like: Picture yourself sitting down to your favourite meal. You've cooked it, and your mouth has been watering, thinking about how delicious it's going to be. You serve it up on the plate and sit down, relaxed with family and friends, to enjoy the food. Your mouth watering is the start of your digestive enzyme production, revving up your stomach acid and signalling to your stomach, gallbladder, and small intestines that food is on its way. You take that first bite, savouring it, chewing to completion (30–40 times), while your friend tells a story about her crazy colleague. As you swallow, your relaxed state (or parasympathetic nervous system) allows your digestive juices to flow, preparing to accept and process that first bite in your acid-filled, churning stomach. After a few bites and a bit of sloshing around, your stomach starts to fill up, and your eating slows. Your brain has been notified that you don't need much more food.

Your partially digested food enters into your small intestine, where it meets with digestive enzymes from the pancreas. Further breakdown of the food occurs here, and then you begin to absorb the nutrients into your bloodstream. Later that night, as you reflect on the company of good friends, feeling satisfied by the entire evening, the digested food is already making its way into the bacterial zone, where the tens of trillions of bacteria in your intestinal tract start to ferment the food and extract more calories. At this point, the bacteria are making food, short-chain fatty acids, to feed your intestinal cells.

Let's imagine, you have the perfect balance of bacteria and therefore you don't experience any bloating, abdominal pain, or weird-smelling gas as you head to bed. Overnight your system keeps doing its thing, bacteria extracting what they need (your cells absorbing nutrients, the lining of the intestines letting only good things through), and your immune system is gatekeeping to ensure that no microbes or whole food particles enter your bloodstream. Your meal finally makes it to the colon with the help of micro contractions, and water is pulled out. When you wake up in the morning, you have a perfect bowel movement and start the cycle over again with breakfast.

Now, this is digestion at its finest, when you are relaxed and having a leisurely dinner. When you have not exposed your body to decades of stress, yo-yo dieting, rounds of antibiotics and other medications, and poor food choices. Many of you probably just read that ideal scenario and thought, *perfect morning bowel movement, flat stomach, no bloating? Yeah, right!* In reality, our digestive system takes a huge hit. And when the digestive system takes a hit, so do our weight loss and health goals.

Here's a brief list of how the gut-weight axis of your body contributes to weight loss resistance, which also makes for a preview of what this chapter holds in store.

- Insufficient fibre and food diversity can lead to poor microbial health, which is associated with weight gain, inflammation, and insulin resistance.
- Nutrient deficiencies arise from insufficient levels of digestive enzymes to properly break down and absorb the food you eat.
- A history of yo-yo dieting can contribute to altered incretin levels. Incretins, which are gut hormones that control your metabolism, help to direct your body as to how much insulin to release and, therefore, fat to store.
- An imbalance of good and bad bacteria alters the release of incretins, affecting weight loss resistance; causes inflammation, affecting insulin resistance and cell health; and alters how many calories your body extracts from what you eat, affecting weight gain.

Take the following two quizzes to help you assess your level of digestive distress. Check yes for all that apply to you.

Digestive Distress Quiz		
Do you experience...?	**Yes**	**No**
cavities		
bad breath		
a thick coating on your tongue		
feeling of heaviness or indigestion		
acid reflux or GERD		
burping frequently		
bloating soon after meals		
fatigue with meals		
headaches or drowsiness with meals		
nausea or vomiting		
bloating with fibre, or worse with fermented foods		
abdominal bloating toward the end of the day		
abdominal pain		
large amounts of, or foul-smelling, gas		
diarrhea		
loose stools		
constipation		
undigested food in your stool		
mucus in your stool		
blood in your stool		
serious hangovers and alcohol intolerance		
poor responses to fat, or high-fat diets		
yeast infections, UTIs		
frequent antibiotic use (>5 times in the last 10 years)		
Eating Pattern Assessment		
Do you...?	**Yes**	**No**
eat quickly		
eat at your desk, computer, or while on the phone		
eat when under stress		
eat similar foods all of the time, i.e., very little variety to meals		
avoid many foods due to sensitivities		
eat at irregular times (including skipping meals)		
cut calories to lose weight		
eat at night		

Do you…?	Yes	No
have, or ever had, binge-eating patterns		
eat foods that bother you (cause bloating, discomfort, joint pain)		
eat refined, processed, or convenience foods >5 times per week		
eat from restaurants frequently (>3 times per week)		

Your Score

If you answered yes to more than eight Digestive Distress questions, then your gut is very likely contributing to your concerns with weight loss and also fatigue, outlook on the world, and experience in your body.

If you answered yes to more than five Eating Pattern Assessment questions, then your food environment really needs work. It is not just *what* you eat but *how* and *when* you eat that contribute to weight loss resistance.

If you scored high on both assessments, you have some work to do. Here's the good news: the solutions offered in this chapter will be key to your success.

The Impacts of a Stressed Digestive System

The state that you eat in is going to have a significant impact beyond the food you eat. As discussed, we have two different nervous systems, one is rest and digest, the other, fight or flight. (See **chapter 4**.) It's no coincidence people of cultures that hold mealtimes sacred experience far fewer digestive issues. Some researchers believe that slowing down to eat meals can even help to control diabetes.

When you remain in a stressed state during meals, your body reacts by producing insufficient digestive enzymes, bacterial imbalances, and you can also get an increase in intestinal permeability, otherwise known as leaky gut. Picture your small intestine as fingerlike projections covered in cheesecloth. Those fingers, known as villi, are where your nutrients are absorbed, and the cheesecloth protects the villi from large pieces of undigested food and large proteins. When large proteins come into contact with the immune system of the villi, a lot of inflammation can result. With leaky gut, the normally tightly woven cheesecloth comes apart, leaving bigger holes and more room for large food proteins to squeeze through.

The most common first sign of leaky gut is inflammatory reactions to foods. Have you ever eaten a food and had no problem with it until one day, after not eating it for a while, that same food gives you aches and pains, possibly a stuffed-up nose, a headache, bloating, diarrhea, or a skin reaction? These could be signs of intestinal permeability. Although there are many things I'll discuss that can help to heal this state, a critical aspect is isolating yourself from stressors—especially perceived stressors during periods when you are eating. When you escape from the stress of the grind, it's also easier to remember to both chew and enjoy your food.

Chewing marks the beginning of the *cephalic phase* of your digestive system. Seeing, smelling, and chewing your food gets the whole system started. You get an increase in your stomach (hydrochloric) acid and digestive enzymes, which work together to break down food and prevent it from being available for all of our bacteria to feed on and overgrow. An overabundance of undigested food results in bloating, an overgrowth of inflammatory bacteria, an overgrowth of your good bacteria in the wrong place (known as small intestinal bacterial overgrowth), gas, and digestive upsets.

Stages of Digestion

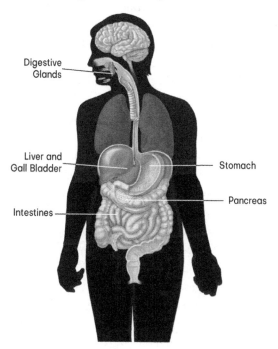

Rested and Relaxed	Rushed and Stressed
Digestive glands – saliva and enzymes produced	Digestive glands – dry mouth, less lubrication and enzymes
Liver/Gallbladder – store sugar in liver. Bile is produced to digest fat, balance bacteria	Liver/Gallbladder – no bile released, liver produces glucose
Stomach – hydrochloric acid and enzymes produced	Stomach – inhibits acid and enzymes
Pancreas – enzymes produced, appropriate insulin and glucagon release to balance blood sugar	Pancreas – decreased enzymes, poor blood sugar control
Intestines – absorption and proper motility occurs	Intestines – poor nutrient absorption, pain, and poor motility

Figure 10. The digestive process starts the moment that food is seen, smelled, or sensed in any way. Digestive enzymes increase and the cascade of hormone release begins. In a rested or relaxed state, left, all the organs are functioning properly and digestion occurs optimally. Effects of eating in a rushed or stressed state, right, impede proper digestion.

The Gut Hormones and Metabolism Control

As food is received in the stomach there should be a decrease in ghrelin, our hunger hormone, signalling that we are getting full. The other satiety hormones, such as CCK and PYY, are released in response to specific nutrients. For example, CCK and PYY are both involved in slowing the rate that food leaves your stomach. These are more strongly regulated by protein and fat; therefore, foods with higher concentrations of these macronutrients can help leave you feeling full longer and support proper food breakdown.[52-54]

Research shows that when satiety hormones are properly regulated, self-control of food consumption and sustained weight loss result.[52,55] Since these hormones are intricately related to the insulin response to food, their function is also important to breaking the fat storage cycle. Working in an obesity research lab, I got exposed to many different mechanisms and theories on how to control weight and diabetes. Gastric bypass surgery, for example, is intended to help morbidly obese people lose weight, thus decreasing their diabetes and other risk factors. But here's what's fascinating: within days of gastric bypass, participants could reduce their medication doses, lower their blood sugar, and regulate their diabetes, even before the weight loss began. You see, gastric bypass works by changing gut hormones, notably the incretins. Incretins are critical to regulating your appetite, blood sugar, and control 50–60% of your insulin release. They are also involved in insulin sensitivity. My big question was, how could they be related to weight loss *resistance*? And do we really need surgery to correct them? The answer to that is one of the breakthroughs in this book.

Gut Hormones and Dieting

At one time or another, the majority of us have yo-yo dieted, i.e., gone on a low-calorie diet, lost weight, increased our calories, and then gained all the weight back, only to start again. When you go on a diet, particularly a low-calorie diet, there's a change in your gut signalling hormones. (In case you were wondering, a low-calorie diet is defined as less than 1,400 kcal. In the long term, this type of diet is a stress on the body. Most women need more than 1,400 kcal just for their organs to work if they were lounging all day! Therefore, if you are eating this little, your body is in starvation mode, especially when you're already stressed or spending hours a week at the gym.)

"STUDIES HAVE SHOWN THAT UP TO ONE YEAR LATER, FOLLOWING A LOW-CALORIE DIET, GUT HORMONES ARE STILL SUPPRESSED, POSSIBLY ACCOUNTING FOR WHY SOME PEOPLE REGAIN WEIGHT LOST, AND OTHERS JUST CAN'T LOSE WEIGHT ON SUBSEQUENT ATTEMPTS."

Table 4. Summary of gut hormones and their functions in weight loss resistance

Name	Hormone Facts	Hormone Functions
Ghrelin	• The "hunger hormone" • Released from the stomach and, to a small degree, the small intestine	• Stimulates hunger and appetite • Promotes fat storage
Leptin	• The "fat stat" • Released from the fat cells	• Controls long-term appetite control and energy expenditure • Controls fat gain and loss
PYY (Peptide-YY)	• Released from the lining of the intestines, the L cells • Released in response to protein or fat	• Regulates the rate of stomach emptying • Increases satiety and nutrient absorption
CCK (Cholecystokinin)	• Released from the lining of the intestines, the I cells • Released in the brain to affect the appetite centres	• Regulates the rate of stomach emptying • Stimulates bile release from the gallbladder to support fat absorption • Stimulates digestive enzymes • Increases satiety and nutrient absorption

Name	Hormone Facts	Hormone Functions
GLP-1 (Glucagon-like peptide-1)	• The main incretin hormone • Released from the lining of the intestines, the L cells • Released in response to sugar or fat	• Regulates the rate of stomach emptying • Increases satiety and nutrient absorption[52,54] • Protects against elevated blood sugar by augmenting insulin release in response to food • Shuts off glucose production in the liver • Increases insulin sensitivity[56]
GIP (Gastric inhibitory peptide)	• Incretin hormone • Released from the lining of the intestines, the K cells • Released in response to sugar	• Increases insulin in response to a meal to protect against high blood sugar • Increases satiety • Increases insulin sensitivity[56]

When you are in a fed state, right after a meal, you have elevated levels of CCK, PYY, leptin, and GLP-1. In contrast, ghrelin, your hungry hormone, drops. Makes sense, right? You just ate, so your brain gets the message that you're full. When you are on a low-calorie diet, however, those fullness and satiety hormones get suppressed, meaning your brain is perpetually told that you don't have enough food. Your gut hormones drop, your body goes into food surveillance mode, and you have to white knuckle it through the day. This makes passing the candy bowl at work or the fast-food joints on your way home feel like a conscious battle.

Here's the astonishing news: studies have shown that up to one year after, following a low-calorie diet, gut hormones are still suppressed, possibly accounting for why some people regain weight lost, and others just can't lose weight on subsequent attempts.[58] Remember, your body is smart; it's primed to save your life and do whatever it takes to pass your genes on to the next generation. The gut hormone system, including incretins, ghrelin, etc., is just one more example of that instinctive protection that occurs.

Now, if you are sitting there, sweating, thinking that you've eternally messed up your body, you're not alone. Never fear, I am here in the trenches with you. We will cover treatment options soon. And no, they don't involve invasive surgery! First, let's consider the important roles of those gut bugs.

How the Good Bugs Turn Bad

There are tens if not hundreds of trillions of bacteria hanging out in and on your body. The gut microbiota—a fancy word for the bacteria, yeast, pathogens, and parasites in your gut—make up a whole other organ of your body. And just like other organs, they help to determine how well we function. These microbiomes can vary widely from one person to the next.

I often tell patients that we have more bacterial DNA in and on our bodies than human DNA. Your gut microbiome has been linked to nearly every chronic disease, like cancer, cardiovascular disease, diabetes, neurological disease, depression, anxiety, liver disease, digestive conditions, and, yes, obesity. If the gut ain't happy, ain't nobody happy! So why aren't we understanding and treating our microbiome imbalances?

That's what we are going to do here! Table 5 provides a summary of the key patterns of bacterial imbalances. You can have one of these patterns, or multiple patterns, and together they have been shown to contribute to weight gain and weight loss resistance.

Table 5: Bacterial imbalances and weight loss resistance

Type of Bacterial Imbalance	Impact on Weight loss
• Bacteroidetes and Firmicutes • Normal bacteria become imbalanced	• Elevated firmicutes contribute to extracting and storing more calories from a meal • Have to eat less to lose weight
• Gram-positive and Gram-negative bacteria • Normal bacteria become imbalanced *or* gram-negative bacterial infection	• Metabolic endotoxemia: inflammation, insulin resistance, weight gain, and altered gut hormones • Contributes to weight loss resistance
• Pathogenic overgrowth/invasion • Normal bacteria and yeast overgrow, causing detrimental symptoms *or* invasive infections	• Inflammation in the digestive system affects satiety, cravings, nutrient deficiencies, and weight gain • The overgrowth or invasion responsible for inflammation affecting the whole body

"YES PEOPLE, A POOP TRANSPLANT COULD BE THE BIKINI PLAN FOR ALL OF US (AND SOME PEOPLE ACTUALLY DO IT!)."

Analyzing and manipulating stool is step number one for any researcher hoping to learn about the impacts of the gut microbiota. Your daily poo is a window into the bug balance of the intestines. Your stool is 25–54% bacterial matter, almost more than the food, toxins, and other waste that leave your body in a daily bowel movement.[59] Researchers have found that these bacterial populations in stool are important. In fact, this research started after a poop transplant from an obese mouse to a lean mouse, and vice versa, was conducted. What do you think happened? If you guessed that the lean mouse got chubby and the chubby mouse became lean (all while eating the same food and doing the same exercise), you would be right! This was the first time that we began to understand how bacterial populations can affect weight gain and weight loss. Yes people, a poop transplant could be the bikini plan for all of us (and some people actually do it!).

Bacteroidetes and Firmicutes

Kidding aside, as the research continued in this area, we came to find patterns in the gut bugs that were present. Although there are trillions and trillions of gut bugs, they can be split into a few different families, or categories. Two of these families are *bacteroidetes* and *firmicutes* and an imbalance of these bugs has been reported consistently in the obesity research. When we are talking about these families of bacteria—and keep in mind, these are still the "good" bacteria, not infections—we are always looking for ratios. When your *firmicutes* are elevated compared to the levels of *bacteroidetes*, you can actually extract more calories from the food that you are eating.[60] This is problematic when you're trying to lose weight because your body can extract more energy, and store more fat, than it should. This is yet another reason why you feel like you aren't eating a lot but the pounds still stay in place.

Gram-Positive and Gram-Negative Bacteria

What I find so much more fascinating, and clinically impactful, is how the groups of bacteria in your gut can affect inflammation levels in your body. When looking at gut bacteria, I find it helpful to think of them as if they were breeds of dog. Dogs are dogs, right? But when you think about it, a Great Dane and a Shih Tzu look quite different. The same is true of their jobs: you would never send a Chihuahua to do the job of a German shepherd police dog. Just as we have the big dogs and the little dogs, the same is true for bacteria. We have some known as *gram-positive* and others as *gram-negative*. The gram-negative bacteria have a sugar coat on the outside that is not so sweet. When you get a lot of these bacteria, you also get a buildup of an inflammatory coat in the gut, known as *lipopolysaccharide (LPS)*. LPS can cross through the thin gut lining, and when it gets into the body in large amounts, problems can ensue. LPS in elevated levels in the bloodstream is known as *metabolic endotoxemia*, which is inflammation that impairs your metabolism. It is a fancy term to tell you that your fat-burning, blood sugar–controlling system has gone out of control. LPS has been directly correlated with weight loss resistance.

Metabolic Endotoxemia

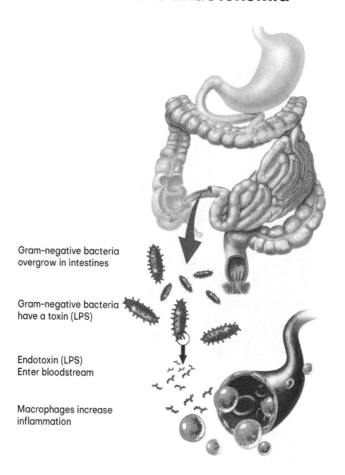

Gram-negative bacteria overgrow in intestines

Gram-negative bacteria have a toxin (LPS)

Endotoxin (LPS) Enter bloodstream

Macrophages increase inflammation

Figure 11. LPS is a sugar found on the outside of gram–negative bacteria that live in the intestine. When LPS gets in the bloodstream it causes white blood cells (macrophages) to increase inflammation and metabolic endotoxemia results from this process.

Gut Bacteria – Metabolic Endotoxemia

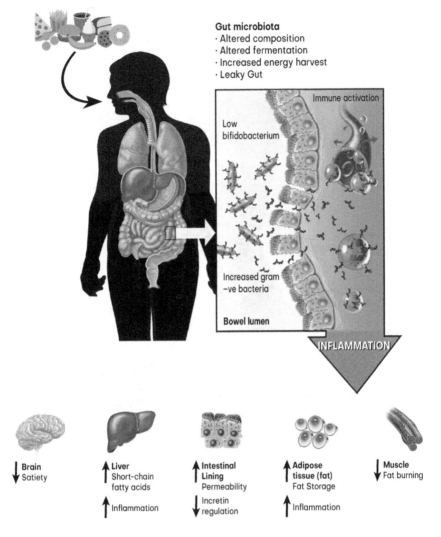

Gut microbiota
· Altered composition
· Altered fermentation
· Increased energy harvest
· Leaky Gut

Immune activation

Low bifidobacterium

Increased gram −ve bacteria

Bowel lumen

INFLAMMATION

| ↓ **Brain** Satiety | ↑ **Liver** Short-chain fatty acids ↑ Inflammation | ↑ **Intestinal Lining** Permeability ↓ Incretin regulation | ↑ **Adipose tissue (fat)** Fat Storage ↑ Inflammation | ↓ **Muscle** Fat burning |

Figure 12. When LPS from gram-negative bacteria leaves your gastrointestinal tract it causes immune activation and an inflammatory response known as metabolic endotoxemia. This inflammation affects your brain through decreasing satiety hormones and affects your liver by altering its fuel sources and increasing inflammation. The lining of your intestinal tract, which is involved in the release of many hormones (see Table 4), becomes leaky and it also increases fat storage and decreases fat burning. LPS creates the perfect environment to foster weight loss resistance.

LPS is a toxin; therefore, it will leave your gut and bind to the receptors on your cells, signalling to your body that there is an internal danger of a threatening infection. When this binding happens, inflammatory signals are activated, and your body becomes primed to fight, just as with the stress system. Inflammation is a type of stress, so your body isn't going to prioritize weight loss when it's inflamed. LPS-induced inflammation also decreases insulin sensitivity, as it changes the way your body stores fat and how much it holds on to. Research has shown animals that eat the exact same food and move the same amount have significantly more weight gain when their blood levels of LPS are elevated.[61,62] The same is true of humans; in fact, when levels of LPS rise, people will gain more weight, and when those levels fall, weight loss becomes easier, insulin sensitivity improves, blood glucose levels improve, and also the health of the liver and the blood vessels improve.[63]

Pathogenic Overgrowth or Invasion

Of course, it's not only the beneficial bacteria and their ratios that have an impact on your metabolism. Overgrowth of normal species, to the point that they cause illness, or other invading infections also have a significant impact on inflammation, the integrity of the gut lining, and metabolic function. Although diagnosis and treatment are far beyond the scope of this book, I do want to explore some signs and symptoms to empower you with an understanding of how these may be affecting you.

SIBO

Small intestinal bacterial overgrowth (SIBO) is becoming increasingly diagnosed. SIBO is exactly what it sounds like, an overgrowth of normal flora in the small intestine. Most of your bacteria should be hanging out and growing in the large intestine, fermenting food, and making food for the intestinal lining (also known as short-chain fatty acids). With stress, a history of gut infections, poor eating habits, poor mitochondrial function, and/or antibiotic use, many gut issues can onset. This includes an underfunctioning of the sweeping system in the gut, known as *migrating motor complexes* that sweep bacteria from the small to large intestine. There can also be issues with the valve between the small and large intestine, which allows for a backflow of sorts. These and many other factors allow for bacteria to grow and develop in the wrong place, which further disturbs digestion, increases inflammation, affects nutrient absorption, energy production, and metabolic function.

SIBO causes a lot of bloating, abdominal discomfort, diarrhea or constipation, and can even cause nausea and joint pain. One of the characteristics of this condition is feeling worse when you eat "health foods" such as fermented foods, or when you take probiotics in a supplement form. Many people with SIBO will try to fix their issues with the conventional wisdom of "add more good bugs," only to end up feeling worse. But in this situation, you're adding more bacteria to the already overfuelled fire; therefore, if you had diarrhea before, that diarrhea will worsen. The same is true of bloating.

Candida or Yeast Overgrowth

Most people in the health and wellness sphere have heard of the candida diet and the life-changing magic of eliminating these bugs. Although I do not believe in the candida diet the way it's currently being recommended, there is something to the fact that so many people feel better on it.

The candida diet is a no sugar, very low-carb diet that's intended to "starve" candida and other yeasts so that they die. It claims to leave you feeling less bloated, less fatigued, less inflamed, and with a plethora of energy and marked weight loss. Although these effects are often true, when carbs are added back to the diet, the issues come right back too. This is because yeast hibernate, they do not starve; they are "smart" and hugely responsive to environmental changes. When yeast are threatened, they will throw up a fuss of inflammation (yes, that's the technical term) and then protect themselves until the food returns, when they come back to life.

All of that said, I highly encourage people with a history of antibiotic use, unrelenting sugar cravings, brain fog, joint pain, and yeast infections or other rashes to explore testing and appropriate treatment for yeast overgrowth. Your waistline, your glucose response, and your inflammation levels will thank you.

Parasites

Parasites can have a huge effect on the body's inflammatory response. They can also induce nutrient deficiencies and even anemia. Indirectly, certain parasites can cause weight gain or weight loss resistance, but that is much less common than yeast, bacterial overgrowth, or species imbalances because parasites often consume your food and frequently cause diarrhea in a way that bacterial or yeast overgrowth alone rarely do. Some parasites can also invade other tissues of the body, having whole body negative effects. If you have been exposed to infected food, untreated water, travelled to warm foreign climates and ended up with diarrhea, flu-like symptoms, joint pain, or new onset anemia, please do not hesitate to march in to your doctor's office and get some parasite testing done. This is discussed more below.

"HERE ARE THE MOST IMPORTANT THINGS TO REMEMBER: YOU WANT A GOOD BALANCE OF BENEFICIAL BACTERIA, NOT TOO MANY AND NOT TOO FEW; YOU WANT ENOUGH BENEFICIAL YEAST, BUT NOT AN OVERGROWTH AND NOT THE NASTY ONES; YOU DON'T WANT PARASITES OR GUT INFECTIONS; AND YOU CERTAINLY DON'T WANT INFLAMMATORY BACTERIA OVERRIDING YOUR SYSTEM, SENDING LPS INTO YOUR BODY, WREAKING HAVOC ON YOUR DIGESTION, METABOLISM, AND ULTIMATELY YOUR WAISTLINE."

Your Diet Did You In

Diet is the most significant factor to account for how we land where we are in relation to a poorly functioning gut. There's a type of diet that we call the Western Diet, which is high in fat, sugar, and processed foods, and low in fibre. Think coffee, a takeout hash brown and egg sandwich meal for breakfast, pop and a hamburger with fries for lunch, a latte and muffin for a snack, and pasta with meat sauce for dinner with some red wine and a slice of chocolate cake for dessert. This may seem like an extreme example to some, but to others it's a reality. This diet has been shown time and time again to mess up those gut bugs.

Your gut bugs are smart; they are also quite adaptive. The good species (those that have more metabolic-boosting, anti-inflammatory properties) need enough fibre, resistant starch, and vegetable and fruit components to thrive. When your diet reflects more of a Western Diet profile different categories of gram-negative bacteria and yeast flourish. They grow, often times out of control, throwing LPS into the system, affecting systemic inflammation, insulin signalling, your body's ability to digest properly and extract nutrients. Many of these species also signal back to the brain, affecting your appetite, cravings (especially sugar cravings), and mood. With this diet we also see an increase in the firmicutes and a decrease in the bacteroidetes, so essentially it's a perfect storm for obesity, insulin resistance, and metabolic syndrome.

High-fat Diet Miracle?

A low-carbohydrate, high-fat diet has been shown in the research to have the best weight loss results for those who are insulin resistant. Given that this was also part of my journey, I jumped on that bandwagon, thinking, this is going to be the thing. To my astonishment at the time, this diet did not go so well for me. Was it that I was eating too many calories, too few calories, working out too much, not enough? I wracked my brain to try to figure out why yet another diet plan, yet another weight loss system (and this one touted everywhere for its health benefits), was actually making me gain weight! I know from working with clients like you, hearing their stories, this happens often, and it's so frustrating.

As I dove into the research, I landed on the explanation: high-fat diets actually pull more LPS from the inside of your gut into the bloodstream! This was the thing that helped to explain the results of so many women.

High-fat diet + gut dysbiosis (gram-negative bacteria) = metabolic endotoxemia, insulin resistance, inflammation, glucose intolerance, and weight gain

This is where I banish the idea of one diet for all people. This is where I shout from the rooftops the need for individualized nutrition plans and a true understanding of physiology before we tell someone they are eating too much and moving too little.

Don't Forget Gut Diversity

Treating the gut is kind of like managing a class of preschoolers in a jungle: there is chaos, frustration, mystery, and just about everything you can think of can go wrong. Just thinking about it is stressful! I don't want you to feel overwhelmed or hopeless; I want you to feel inspired. I am giving you a ton of information, and also purposefully leaving things out to avoid completely overwhelming you. (Maybe those things will be for my next book.)

Here are the most important points to remember: you want a good balance of beneficial bacteria, not too many and not too few; you want enough beneficial yeast, but not an overgrowth and not the nasty ones. You don't want parasites or gut infections, and you certainly don't want inflammatory bacteria overriding your system, sending LPS into your body, wreaking havoc on your digestion, metabolism, and ultimately your waistline. So what else could there be? Well, variety for one thing.

Not only do we need to look at the types of bacteria in the gut, but we also need to consider their variety. Just like a jungle would not function with five species of plants, the gut cannot thrive and be the peaceful anti-inflammatory space we would like it to be without a wide diversity of bugs. We need trillions of bugs from millions of different strains and species to achieve gut harmony. This is no easy feat today, as we all need different food, fibre, colourful fruits and vegetables, sugar but not too much, hormones but not too many, proper liver function, and minimal toxin exposure. Above all things though, to have a lean, healthy, bloat-free gut, we need to consider antibiotics, the medications you get for every sore throat, earache, and chest infection.

Perhaps you took countless antibiotics as a child and possibly have given them to your children, if you're a parent. Antibiotics are now pervasive. They are found in our water supply and fed to livestock through their feed to increase weight gain; therefore, these drugs affect the water we drink and the meat we eat. Let me be clear: antibiotics save lives and should not be avoided in cases of serious infection. However, we should be using them more conservatively, because antibiotics have been shown to be the number one diversity-destroying substance humans have encountered. Not only do they have long-standing impacts on our digestive symptoms and inflammation, but they can also affect weight. The agricultural industry permits many questionable practices to boost livestock growth rates; the most pertinent in this context is low-level antibiotic exposure.[64,65] I would go so far as to say if you have had recent or regular antibiotic exposure, and you experienced weight gain or weight loss resistance, then supporting your gut diversity is the place to start assessing the root cause of your weight loss resistance.

Diagnostic Tools for Gut Health

Although I can lay out every quiz possible to help you diagnose your gut issues, the reality is that gut imbalances, infections, and inflammation are the ultimate doppelgängers. Because I have often been surprised by the results of testing that come into my office, I think testing is a good idea.

However, there is no perfect gut microbiome testing today. With a quick online search, you will be bombarded with research and opinions for and against all types of testing. In my opinion, this is because we are just coming into an age where we are understanding the importance of the gut and how to measure species and effects. There are also species that we may never know, simply because our technology doesn't know how to pick them up, or because they don't come out in our stool. Below is a starter guide for testing, and things to consider when speaking to your doctor or buying a test.

Ova and Parasite Testing

Ova and parasite testing, or O&P testing, is the standard poop culture. This testing is a measurement of visible parasites or their eggs in your poop. It needs to be done over three samples, on three days, from different parts of your poop because parasites grow, shed, and procreate on different cycles.

Stool Culture

Stool cultures are often done alongside O&P testing to see if any microbes (bacteria, yeast, or pathogens) grow and can be detected while being cultured. This test has many limitations though, as most of our microbes are anaerobic, meaning they do not live and grow well if exposed to oxygen.

GI Pathogen Panel

GI pathogen testing can be as comprehensive or simple as the clinician or lab requests. It's a type of testing that picks up the DNA and RNA (genetic components) of the bacteria present through a lab technique known as PCR. It's the gold standard for many pathogens as they may or may not be growing or living in that specific stool sample, but chances are pieces of them or their DNA can be found. GI pathogen tests are often recommended if you have a parasite, virus, or pathogenic microbe, but only specific labs will offer whole microbiome screens.

Bacterial Sequencing Tools

The world of gut microbiome sequencing is getting to be very competitive. Every laboratory, research group, and doctor wants a piece of the pie. Although this is great for patient care, it means that technology is always changing, every company says that it's better and more accurate, and it's more confusing than ever to know what to do.

The main thing to consider when thinking about testing is what you are hoping to achieve. If you think you have a parasite, or some type of gut infection, and you have had a history of antibiotics use, you may want to consider one of the tests that explore PCR DNA/RNA tests of the microbiome species, along with testing for O&P and markers of inflammation. Stool culture tests may also claim to provide information on species, diversity, inflammation, and O&P (although the accuracy of these tests has been brought into question more in recent years). As we cannot culture many species in the gut, researchers are suggesting that just running a culture test may not provide the most extensive information on the balance between inflammatory and anti-inflammatory species, bacterial diversity, or ratios such as the balance of firmicutes to bacteroidetes. However, these tests are often accurate for stool markers of inflammation, basic information about pathogenic species, and serious overgrowths. They are also less expensive, which is a perk. If finances are an obstacle but you truly feel there may be issues, even if your primary care testing was negative, culture or urine testing may provide more information.

Urine Organic Acids

Urinary organic acids testing has been done for years in the autism, fatigue, and chronic disease world, but it's just now becoming more mainstream. Although the full organic acids profile is very comprehensive in its view of mitochondrial health, neurotransmitters, and nutrient deficiencies, there's now a subsection of the test that runs only the microbial aspect as opposed to the whole test. The Microbial Organic Acids Test (MOAT) investigates the breakdown products of yeast, general markers of bacteria, bacterial overgrowth, and some pathogenic inflammatory species in the clostridia family. This test does not give insight into the microbial diversity, types of species, inflammatory status, or the ratio of the firmicutes to bacteroidetes. What it does provide is an overview of what's happening throughout the gut, not just in the large intestine or colon. This test is also accurate for yeast overgrowth, whereas many of the other culture tests have not been established to be consistently accurate. If you suspect yeast overgrowth, want an overview of your microbial balance, or struggle with chronic fatigue, burnout, or other neurological issues, you may want to explore the MOAT or Organic Acids Test (OAT) test, respectively.

Go for the Gut

If the information in this chapter does not motivate you to take your gut health seriously, I don't know what will. It can be the missing piece, or at least a critical piece, of the whole equation for you. In order to address the gut issues that may be dogging you, I want you to challenge yourself to think big picture. The unfortunate reality is that there's no one supplement that is going to change your life when the ultimate goal is weight regulation. But you know that, you've tried them! Probiotics can be hugely powerful when it comes to changing the immune state of your gut, improving bloating, gas, constipation, diarrhea, even hormone balance, but they alone have not shown clinically impactful changes on weight loss. Why? Well because, it's not about one type of bacteria, it's about diversity, ratios, inflammation, and pathogen overgrowth, the food you eat, and the nutrient power and timing of that food. So if you are having significant issues with digestion, please, by all means, get testing, address those potential overgrowths, infections, and the like. Without that, you will likely continue to struggle even with the following suggestions. But when you are done testing, I urge you to hop over here and set yourself up for lifelong gut health, to kick the inflammation and the metabolic endotoxemia, to regulate those hormones, and to lose the weight and get your vitality back!

Prebiotics versus Probiotics

Some of you may have been surprised to read that supplementing probiotic pills does not have a direct impact on weight loss resistance. Throughout this chapter, I've made the case that changing the gut microbiome does have an impact, so now what can you do to support your good bugs? It's critical to understand the difference between prebiotics, probiotic supplements, and fermented food.

Probiotics are the actual beneficial bacteria whereas prebiotics are the food for that bacteria. Probiotics include the bifidobacteria, lactobacillus, and beneficial yeast species. These can be taken in a pill or a powder and are now often added to yogurts or drinks. For instance, lactobacillus species are added to certain yogurts. Natural probiotics also can be obtained from naturally fermented food, such as sauerkraut, kimchi, kombucha, and natural yogurts, which have a whole range of bacteria and yeast that can add to the diversity of the gut microbiome.

Prebiotics, the food source for the bacteria, are found not only in the list of foods to the right, but also probiotics can be packaged with prebiotics to help feed the bacteria when they reach your gut. The prebiotics are different fibres, starches, and sugars, known as fructooligosaccharides, that the bacteria eat up. They occur in our food, can be supplemented on their own, and are often added to foods. Their weight loss benefits are discussed below.

Prebiotic Foods
• Chia seed
• Flax seed
• Acacia gum
• Guar gum
• Potato starch
• Inulin
• Chicory root
• Jerusalem artichoke
• Onion
• Garlic
• Leek
• Dandelion greens

When and How You Eat

Meal Timing

There is an overwhelming amount of conflicting information and research on food timing. Is breakfast the most important meal of the day? Should you skip it? Should you eat two meals, three meals, or five meals per day? And these concerns don't even touch *what* should be consumed at those times! Aside from circadian rhythm considerations, i.e., eating during daylight hours, each of us will have individual meal timing needs. For example, therapeutic or intermittent fasting is all the rage these days in the health community. One of the most common ways it's described is as a sixteen-hour fast with an eight-hour eating window. Eating in this manner requires most people to skip either breakfast or dinner, eating two larger meals and potentially a snack during that time. This diet is touted to reset insulin signalling, clear brain fog, reset cravings, and help you to effortlessly achieve the body weight of your dreams. Although I might have exaggerated on that last point, you may have heard similar things in the marketing of this lifestyle.

Intermittent fasting, or IF, is something that I use regularly as a therapeutic tool. Great benefits can be achieved with this protocol, *but* if you are stressed out, not sleeping, and your adrenals are not producing cortisol at the proper times of day, then my experience is that IF will only put you in a deeper stressed state, and we need to start by addressing the pre-existing stressors first. Some studies have shown that skipping breakfast can alter the production of satiety hormones, causing the consumption of more calorically dense foods and more binge-type eating later in the day. If you find yourself falling face first into carbs when you skip your early morning eats then it's not for you.

Another study showed that in those living with type 2 diabetes, skipping breakfast can decrease the gut hormone GLP-1 response to food, increase the glucose response to a food, and induce insulin resistance throughout the day.[66] Interestingly, for those with diabetes, eating two meals per day, focusing on breakfast and lunch, did not seem to have negative effects on gut hormones but did improve weight loss.[67] This just goes to show that IF does not equal simply skipping breakfast, and reinforces the importance of the circadian rhythm on eating in certain conditions.

I stand strongly for restricting your eating window, and whether you eat your meals within a twelve-hour window or an eight-hour window, and whether that window is from 8:00 a.m. to 4:00 p.m. or 12:00 p.m. to 8:00 p.m. is going to be personal. It's going to depend on where your circadian rhythm is now, and where we need to move it to. It's going to depend on your stress, hormones, inflammation and insulin levels. One thing is certain though: if you are eating from 8:00 a.m. to

12:00 a.m. and snacking at all hours, we have work to do. Your gut hormones, gut bacteria, and digestive system need to follow a circadian rhythm.

Take Action
I bet the thought of skipping a meal, going without snacking, or restricting your eating window has stirred resistance in some of you. I know I had strong opinions about it at first too. So wherever you are, let's adopt a growth mindset and take the first step toward cutting out snacks, aiming first for three meals per day within a 12-hour eating window. Then push on toward 10, nine, or eight hours, if you feel well doing it. There's no need to get dizzy, anxious, hangry, or obsessive about it. *Play with it.* We'll go over this again when we put the whole plan together.

Chewing

I've mentioned the importance of chewing earlier in this chapter, so this serves as a reminder. Chewing is critical to trigger the digestive juices, increasing stomach acid levels and enzymes and proper motility, or movement, in the gut. (This activity is significant if you don't want a bacterial overgrowth or dysbiosis.) Chewing also stimulates the release of gut hormones, GIP and GLP-1, which are critical to the regulation of glucose and insulin sensitivity. Finally, if you find you end up too full at the end of a meal, or alternatively, seem to eat all day and never feel truly full, make sure you are getting those bites in, because chewing also stimulates our satiety hormones, letting the body know you are full and ready to carry on with your day. These hormones, PYY and CCK, not only have effects on your feeling of fullness, but they are also just the start of the digestion cascade. Without proper signalling, you can perpetually feel hungry and on the lookout for food. This has been shown to contribute to weight regain and yo-yo dieting.

Your goal here: 20 to 40 chews per bite. Burn those calories! (Chewing uses a muscle, right? It must be classed as exercise!) If even after a good meal in a calm place and ample chewing you still aren't feeling full, it's time to dive into more fibre!

Breaking Down the Diet for Gut Health

By now, you now know when to eat and how to eat, so it's time to explore what to eat. When it comes to eating for gut health, the information can feel overwhelming. But it doesn't have to. The diet I have outlined for you will increase the good bugs, lower inflammation, and support weight loss. Win-win-win!

"PREBIOTICS, SUCH AS INULIN, ACACIA, AND RESISTANCE STARCH LIKE POTATO STARCH, HELP TO INCREASE GLP-1, INCREASE INSULIN SENSITIVITY, LOWER GLUCOSE, AND HELP YOU TO LOSE WEIGHT."

Benefits of Fibre

Fibre is the first category of nutrients you need to consider. Did you know that our ancestors ate 40–50 g of fibre per day? Today we are lucky if we get 15 g, which is less than one-third of what you need. I am a bit of a fibre and prebiotic junkie because these components have so many benefits. Fibre helps to balance our hormones, bind and eliminate toxins, and keep the poop flowing. Certain fibres also feed your gut bacteria, prebiotics, and change your gut hormones. Soluble fibres or resistance starches are the preferred fuel for many beneficial gut bacterial species. As a general rule, when your bacteria eat fibre, they produce short-chain fatty acids, which serve as fuel to the cells of the gut lining, known as *enterocytes*. These enterocytes protect the integrity of the lining, preventing leaky gut, inflammation, and food intolerances. The short-chain fatty acids also signal for the proper release of gut hormones.[61,68,69] This is one of the ways that prebiotics, such as inulin, acacia, and resistance starch like potato starch, help to increase GLP-1, increase insulin sensitivity, lower glucose, and help you to lose weight.

Much of the research on fibres changing bacterial population includes inulin, inulin type fructans, acacia gum, and resistance starches such as potato starch. The fibres listed above have specifically been shown to help balance out the firmicutes to bacteroidetes ratio, skewing the bacterial population to reflect more of a lean person's poop. Increasing dietary fibre in general also increases anti-inflammatory species of bacteria such as the bifidobacteria.[69–71] The addition of dietary fibre also fosters diversity of the gut microbiome, which is protective against many diseases, far beyond considering your weight loss goals.

Among these fibres, I have mentioned acacia a few times. If you have a sensitive gut, it may be the one to start with. Acacia gum, purchased as a powder at the health food store, is one of the more gentle prebiotic fibres that, when consumed at 30 g per day, can help increase diversity of beneficial bacteria and it can help you to lose body fat, without the bloating and gas that may come with some other bacterial fuels.[72]

If you have ever taken a prebiotic or a probiotic, or increased your dietary fibre and felt awful, this section is for you. First, when you are adding more fuel to your bacteria's fire, especially when they are not accustomed to it, they get excited! This can show up as transient gas, bloating, and some poop changes for three to five days. The same thing can happen when you add new types of bacteria; these can cause a little bit of a battle between the bugs (they get territorial), and the same symptoms can occur. This should all be transient though. When it is not, or when the symptoms are severe, with diarrhea, pain, brain fog, low mood, or an increase in the inflammation in your body, then you should be digging deeper. Whenever this happens I am concerned about a gut pathogen, or alternatively—and commonly—SIBO. This is your warning: if you are having prolonged or significant symptoms, please don't tough it out. Listen to your body and stop. You may have found your underlying issue.

One of the benefits I find the most fascinating is that proper intake of fibre can actually protect your body from metabolic endotoxemia. Remember the discussion of LPS, that coat on the outside of certain types of bacteria, and how it increases inflammation, decreases insulin sensitivity, messes with your hormones, and keeps you feeling fat, fatigued, and achy? Well, all that you have to do, my friend, is jack up fibre consumption to start the healing process! There is no consensus in the research about the dose of inulin to lower circulating LPS and help to heal your gut. Doses range from 3 g to 30 g. This is likely because the human microbiome is so incredibly diverse. The amount of gram-negative LPS–containing bacteria in my gut will be different from yours and vice versa. Many also experience SIBO, dysbiosis, and yeast overgrowths that are not accounted for in the research.

In any case, fibre can be powerful. Just one of the many studies showed that a mix of inulin and a fermentable sugar, oligofructans, at 16 g per day was able to increase anti-inflammatory bacteria and decrease the amount of circulating LPS in women. Small changes in fat mass and inflammation were seen.[71] Yet another example showed a 35.9% decrease in insulin resistance, a 35.6% decrease in hs-CRP (a marker of inflammation), and a 27.9% decrease in LPS, with only 10 g of inulin daily over eight weeks![73] Outside of the fibre world, resistant starch, such as potato starch at 10 g per day, can decrease insulin 29.36%, insulin resistance by 32.85% and lower endotoxin 25.00%.[74] Worth a try? I think so!

Take Action
Inulin, acacia, and potato starch can be found at any health food store. Powder forms easily dissolve in smoothies or water, but remember they need to be consumed cold! No adding to soups or stews because the heat changes the way the bacteria can use them.

Dietary and supplemented fibres not only have a positive impact on gut bacteria, but they can also improve satiety. Fibre in general, including the ones listed above, and other powerful ones known as glucomannan/konjac-mannan, or PGX, help to control appetite, lower the glucose response to foods, and keep you feeling full.[75] If you have ever seen or used a fibre like glucomannan, you will also know how powerfully this fibre can suck up water. You do not want to leave this sitting too long in your glass because it can become very thick and gelatinous, which can be a challenge to finish. For this reason, having this fibre 30 minutes before meals has been shown to help to achieve weight loss.

Polyphenols

Have you ever heard of a superfood? Blueberries, acai, chocolate, green tea, coffee, and pomegranates have all become labelled superfoods for their health-promoting effects. Supporting glucose regulation, heart health, and anti-inflammatory effects are some of the touted benefits. These superfoods have been grouped together because of their polyphenolic components. Polyphenols are chemicals that a plant produces to protect itself, and just as there are different types of bacteria, there are also different types of polyphenols, often characterized as flavonoids, phenolic acids, stilbenes, and lignans. This is important to know if you're ever looking further into the area, or get confused about the terminology, but the whole category of polyphenols has weight loss, anti-inflammatory, insulin-sensitizing benefits.

The functions of polyphenols are divided into four main categories. First and foremost, polyphenols can decrease metabolic endotoxemia by decreasing the movement of LPS from your gut into your bloodstream (see Figure 11, page 115). Second, they work to decrease inflammation in the body. Third, polyphenols can feed specific types of bacteria as if they were fibre, increasing the bifidobacteria populations, which also improves insulin signalling and weight regulation.[76-78] This may be one of the mechanisms by which polyphenols can increase gut hormones like GLP-1. Finally, polyphenols may interfere with carbohydrate breakdown and glucose absorption, reducing the impact of the carbs you eat on your blood sugar response.[79] Essentially, you can tolerate more carbohydrates and dietary sugars because the polyphenols act as shields, blocking them from having a dramatic effect on your insulin and sugar.

There is no good answer as to which are the best polyphenols because, again, it's more about the amount and the diversity of polyphenols than using one in isolation. Coffee, green tea, cocoa, red wine, blueberry, quercetin, cinnamon, and resveratrol for instance, all have supportive characteristics. The key point to remember with polyphenols—and even prebiotics and fibre to some extent—is that I'm not talking about a pill here. The goal is for you to eat foods that are rich in these things. That is where the benefits come with diabetes, insulin sensitivity, and weight loss. In isolation, none of these ingredients offers significant benefits. Think about it: if you pop a pill of blueberry extract while eating a meal from McDonald's, it isn't going to take you far. This is where I promote working your way into a diet that includes 30–45 g of fibre per day, and at least 2,000 mg (2 g) of polyphenolics from the fruits, vegetables, drinks, and spices high in polyphenols in Table 6 .[80] This is the diet we need for gut health and metabolic health.

Table 6. Polyphenol chart

| Food | Food group | Polyphenols | | |
		Content (mg/100g)	Per serving (aim for 2,000 mg/day)	Size (approx.)
Black elderberry	Fruits	1359	1359	2/3 cup
Chestnut	Seeds	1215	1215	2/3 cup
Lowbush blueberry	Fruits	836	836	2/3 cup
Blackcurrant	Fruits	758	758	2/3 cup
Highbush blue-berry	Fruits	560	560	2/3 cup
Hazelnut	Seeds	495	495	2/3 cup
Pecan nut	Seeds	493	493	2/3 cup
Plum	Fruits	377	377	2/3 cup
Sweet cherry	Fruits	274	274	2/3 cup
Globe artichoke heads	Vegetables	260	260	1 cup
Blackberry	Fruits	260	260	2/3 cup
Strawberry	Fruits	235	235	2/3 cup
Red raspberry	Fruits	215	215	2/3 cup
Coffee	Non-alcoholic beverages	214	214	2 cups
Prune	Fruits	194	194	2/3 cup
Almond	Seeds	187	187	2/3 cup
Red wine	Alcoholic beverages	101	176.8	1 six-ounce glass

Food	Food group	Polyphenols		
		Content (mg/100g)	Per serving (aim for 2,000 mg/day)	Size (approx.)
Black grape	Fruits	169	169	2/3 cup
Red onion	Vegetables	168	168	½ c
Apple	Fruits	136	136	½ medium
Peppermint, dried	Seasonings	11960	119.6	1 tsp.
Spinach	Vegetables	119	119	3 cups
Shallot	Vegetables	113	113	½ cup
Black olive	Vegetables	569	81.3	6 olives
Cloves	Seasonings	15188	75.9	1 tsp.
Pure pomegranate juice	Non-alcoholic beverages	66	66	100 mL
Peach	Fruits	59	59	½ medium
Dark chocolate (70%)	Cocoa products	1664	166.4	1 square (10 g)
Capers	Seasonings	654	54.5	1 tsp.
Green olive	Vegetables	346	49.4	6 olives
Broccoli	Vegetables	45	45	½ cup
Black bean	Seeds	59	44.3	½ cup
Red currant	Fruits	43	43	2/3 cup
White bean	Seeds	51	38.3	½ cup
Cocoa powder	Cocoa products	3448	34.5	1 tsp.
Apricot	Fruits	34	34	1 small
Asparagus	Vegetables	29	29	¾ cup chopped, 6 large spears
Walnut	Seeds	28	28	2/3 cup
Red lettuce	Vegetables	23	23	3 cups
Extra virgin olive oil	Oils	62	8.9	1 Tbsp.
Black tea	Non-alcoholic beverages	102	4.1	1 tsp.
Green tea	Non-alcoholic beverages	89	3.6	1 tsp.
Most culinary herbs and herbal teas	Herbs	100	5	1 tsp.

Significant changes to your fibre and polyphenol intake need to be made gradually. Even if you are a healthy eater, you likely have room to improve in these categories. I often recommend that people start by increasing only 5–10 g of fibre per week, and aim to increase polyphenols to 2,000 mg over one week. This allows time for your gut bacteria to adjust, balance out, and become friendly with the new food choices, as opposed to throwing you into digestive distress.

Cautionary Note on Red Wine

Yes, I did mention red wine in the polyphenol section. The resveratrol component of red wine is indeed a lovely source of polyphenols, when used in moderation. Before choosing a glass of your favourite red as your source of polyphenols for the day, I'd be remiss if I didn't point out that although red wine has many health-promoting benefits, if you have gut inflammation, it may do more harm than good. Alcohol, including red wine, has been shown to increase intestinal hyperpermeability, or leaky gut, shuttling LPS right into your bloodstream.[81] This is partly why we have hangovers, and partly why alcohol consumption actually slows your metabolism.

"WHAT PEOPLE OFTEN FORGET WHEN THEY'RE DIETING IS, *IT'S NOT THE FOOD'S FAULT*, THERE IS NO BAD FOOD OR GOOD FOOD. *IT'S YOUR BODY THAT NEEDS TO CHANGE*, AND WE CAN USE FOOD CHOICES TO HELP BRING ABOUT THOSE CHANGES."

Level Up with Supplements

So far, I've addressed diet and lifestyle changes as the main way to effect changes to the gut microbiome, metabolic endotoxemia, and gut hormone responses. I firmly believe that such changes always have, and always will, start with food. After years of trying to use different food-based diets to lose weight, to no avail, it can be completely disheartening to think about one more diet change. I get that, believe me.

I know that you have probably tried low carb, no carb, high protein, vegetarian, low fat, moderation, or a combination of these. What people often forget when they're dieting is, it's not the food's fault, there is no bad food or good food. It's your body that needs to change, and we can use food choices to help bring about those changes. Food is not just about macronutrients, and it certainly isn't calorie-cutting that's going to help you reach your goals. We need to get used to thinking of food in terms of quality and nutrient density and how it will affect our cells, our bacteria, and our hormones. That is why this chapter and the next are supplement-poor and diet-rich. This is also why I have a whole chapter that will walk you through a true food and lifestyle change, so that you too can lose the weight you want to lose, keep it off, increase your energy, balance your hormones, heal your gut, and feel like you are living fully again.

For now, I will give you the supplement pieces of the puzzle, with the warning that I do not want you to run out and buy everything. Keep experimenting with foods first! If you have made it to the end of week two of the plan and you're still feeling like your weight loss and digestion need more support, then here are some options to try.

Apple Cider Vinegar and Digestive Enzymes

A strong digestive system starts before the food digestion process even begins. Earlier in this chapter, I discussed the cephalic phase of digestion, where stomach acid starts to be secreted and digestive enzymes are signalled to start flowing. Adequate levels of these are critical for proper gut microbial balance and appropriate gut and satiety hormone signalling. When you have enough stomach acid, it also functions to protect you from other pathogenic invaders. Have you ever gotten awful food poisoning whereas someone else at the table, eating the same thing, had no symptoms at all? This could have been because they had enough acid to kill off the organisms. Stomach acid and enzymes also prevent undigested food from entering into the "bacteria rich zones" of your intestine where the bacteria can eat that leftover food and, therefore, overgrow.

Why would someone have low levels of stomach acid or digestive enzymes? Well, stressors, distracted eating, and inadequate chewing play big roles! If you bloat after you eat, feel indigestion, or have undigested food in your stool, it's time to support that system. Given that we've already covered chewing and how you eat, let's dive right into my favourite support, apple cider vinegar (ACV), and other enzyme supplements.

ACV can stimulate the production of stomach acid and enzymes, and as we will discuss in the next chapter, it can also affect gut hormones and insulin release. For now though, think of that mouth-watering feeling you get when you eat bitter foods. That *salivation* is the start of your acid and enzymes secretion. One to two tsp. of ACV in a small amount of water, taken 10-15 minutes before each meal can help to support digestion. This is a gentle way to increase acid and enzymes. Caution though: if you get a burning in your stomach or acid reflux when starting ACV, you may have enough stomach acid; therefore, looking into other causes of your digestive issues is important.

(Note of caution: if ACV is greatly helping your digestion and you plan to use it long term then it is advisable to drink it through a straw. Some state that it can have an impact on tooth enamel.)

Digestive enzymes can be used if the ACV helps but does not quite fix the problem. There are hundreds of digestive enzymes on the market and finding one that is well rounded is key. The things to look for in a digestive enzyme include:

- Amylase: breaks down carbohydrates known as amylose
- Lipase: breaks down fats
- Protease: breaks down protein
- Bromelain (from pineapple): supports proper acid levels and general digestion
- Papain (from papaya): supports proper acid levels and general digestion
- Cellulase: breaks down the fibre cellulose
- Pepsin: supports protein breakdown in the stomach
- Betaine HCl: stomach acid, used only if you have low acid levels (This can be tested with ACV first.)

Digestive enzymes can be taken with your first bite of a meal and should help to lower bloating and help you feel full but not sluggish after meals. Every few weeks it's important to take a break from the enzymes to see if your own body's production has increased to sufficient levels. As you change your diet and address sleep, stress, and your circadian rhythm, it's very common for your body to pick up the slack and start making its own acid and enzymes again.

Berberine

Berberine is a natural plant alkaloid that has diverse uses in natural medicine, mainly as an anti-diabetic, anti-inflammatory, and lipid-lowering agent. One of the most interesting groups of studies on berberine suggests that it has an equal insulin-sensitizing effect to metformin, which is a pharmaceutical diabetes medication.[82] We now know that berberine also helps to modulate GLP-1 and gut hormones through its action on the gut microbiome.[83] (As a bonus, it can also decrease brain fog and support neurological health.)

Symptoms of bloating, gas, constipation, and even immense sugar cravings can tip you off that gut microbial imbalances may be at the root of your weight loss resistance. Berberine is one supplement that has an impact on all of these symptoms. Another scenario in which berberine can be used is when your blood glucose or insulin levels are higher than the ideal ranges that I have listed in appendix A. If you have not had recent blood work done, or have no digestive concerns, berberine may not be the supplement for you.

The dosage of berberine is 300–500 mg, three times per day. This should be used for a maximum of three months, as it has a powerful impact on the gut bacteria.

Omega-3 Fatty Acids

Omega-3 fatty acids hold so many benefits, including decreasing inflammation via reducing metabolic endotoxemia and reducing LPS.[84] The most highly anti-inflammatory omega-3 fatty acid is eicosapentaenoic acid (EPA). At 1,500 mg of EPA per day, changes in inflammation, insulin sensitivity, and glucose signalling occur. The DHA content has also been shown to be important; therefore, aiming for at least 500 mg of DHA is advisable both for brain health and weight loss.

In addition to weight loss resistance, omega-3 fatty acids have been shown to reduce brain fog, depression, and anxiety and many skin conditions, including acne, eczema, psoriasis, and dry skin. The skin and brain are mainly water and fat; the same is true of all of our cells. This is why good-quality fats are key!

Long-term use of anti-inflammatory omega-3 fatty acids is safe for the majority of the population, although it is still good to check in with a healthcare provider. If you are on any blood-thinning medications or have a history of blood clots, then you sit in the minority and should not take this supplement.

The Finally Lose it Gut Review

- Digestion starts from the moment you think about food and is controlled by the brain, which is why having the complete smell, see, taste, and chew experience with food is critical to healthy digestion.
- Your digestive system is so much more than a poop machine. The nutrients absorbed here, the hormones released, and the immune system that sits along this tract have significant implications for whole body inflammation and insulin sensitivity.
- The gut hormones most critical to weight loss resistance include satiety/fullness hormones (PYY, CCK, ghrelin, GLP-1) and the incretins (GLP-1, GIP), which are highly involved in blood glucose control and insulin release.
- Inflammation in the gastrointestinal tract can come from many sources: intestinal hyperpermeability, food sensitivities, and, commonly, imbalances between the types of bacteria and pathogens present in the gut. An imbalance between the firmicutes and the bacteroidetes has been associated with weight gain, as has an increase in LPS-producing bacteria, which are involved in metabolic endotoxemia.
- The main insults to gut and bacterial health include eating in a hurried, stressed state; yo-yo dieting; taking antibiotics; insufficient fibre or polyphenol consumption; and overeating a Western Diet.
- Diet, meal timing, and increasing the amount of fibre (to 45 g daily) and polyphenols (to 2,000 mg daily) have all proven to support proper gut hormone signalling, balance bacteria, and lower inflammation. Together these support insulin signalling, weight loss, mental clarity, and reduce bloating, gas, and regulate the bowels.
- If you need more support beyond what this chapter recommends to reach your weight loss goals, appropriate GI testing and supplements may be needed.

BE **STUBBORN** ABOUT YOUR GOALS. BE **FLEXIBLE** ABOUT YOUR METHODS.

—ANONYMOUS

6

THE FAT-BURNING BLOCKER

Insulin and Insulin Resistance

nsulin is a hormone released by the pancreas in response to consumption of specific macronutrients, namely carbohydrates and proteins. Insulin performs a necessary function in the body, binding to insulin receptors on cells and taking sugar from your bloodstream to your liver, muscles, and fat cells for storage. Too much insulin, however, leads to too much fat storage and not enough fat burning. This is often referred to as being in a state of sugar burning versus fat burning. Insulin also has significant effects on the brain, skin health, reproduction, and cravings. Proper insulin release and proper insulin receptor function, or sensitivity, have a direct impact on whole body health. The problem is that very few people function optimally in this area. Hyperinsulinemia (too much insulin released) and insulin resistance are the final physiological blocks we'll explore in weight loss resistance. Insulin resistance is a protective state in which the body stops listening to the signals insulin sends. This inappropriate insulin response traps your fat in your fat cells, your blood sugar is not properly controlled, and your body tells your brain not to let go of a single pound. This is why diets haven't worked for you! You have seen throughout this book that insulin release and insulin resistance are critical pieces to weight loss resistance. This is the chapter where we dive into the details of that relationship.

Mary Ann was the quintessential example of an insulin resistant woman. At age 35 she was a busy mom of two and director at a local financial company. She was highly motivated to achieve in all aspects of her life, but her weight and her health were two areas where she just wasn't able to see the benefits of the work she was putting in. Mary Ann had always been on the chubbier side. Everyone in her family seemed to have a similar build, but she was generally able to keep her weight under control with diet and exercise. Recently, her standard strategies weren't working, and she could not figure out why. Mary Ann's weight crept up with each pregnancy and continued to creep up—5 lbs with every holiday and 1–2 lbs every month outside of that. She had jumped back on her plan, counting points, eating five to six small meals a day, increasing her lean protein and low-fat snacks. The only thing that she wasn't able to add back in was the rigorous (and borderline abusive) workout routine that she would follow during her pre-baby phase.

Her goal was to whittle her middle, but instead it continued to grow and expand. Strangely, she thought, her legs seemed to be the only body part of her body that she was able to maintain in good form. She felt as if the increasing weight just stuck to her stomach, arms, and back. With two babies and a demanding job, she was resorting to an even lower calorie approach but hunger and complete exasperation with the process often led to late-night snack attacks, as her body capitalized on moments of weakness.

When Mary Ann came to see me, she was multiple dress sizes above where she felt most comfortable. She was losing confidence in her body, in herself, and in her food choices. Mary Ann had recently had a panel of blood work done and everything had come back "normal." She was doing all the "right things," and was apparently healthy. So what was up?

Together, we established that her weight loss resistance was related to her stressed and overwhelmed state and staying awake all hours to accomplish everything she wanted to. She was also eating at all hours of the night to keep herself awake and motivated. Beyond that, Mary Ann was eating low-fat, high-carb meals and snacking throughout the day, which, when combined with a genetic predisposition, set her up for metabolic chaos. Even though she was following what the current diet paradigm suggested, she was a victim to the system and needed to understand her body, and insulin function, in a whole new light.

Although Mary Ann was a classic physical picture of insulin resistance, gaining weight in her belly and back, we still wanted to quantify just how insulin resistant she was. When I ran my blood work, her inflammatory markers and insulin were far from normal. Mary Ann had a fasting insulin level three times what is ideal, locking her in fat storage mode. At the end of the two-hour testing, her insulin also remained high, meaning her snacks throughout the day were just putting the padlock on those fat cells. All of this, despite "normal" results from her previous physical.

I treated Mary Ann rather aggressively. I gave her three weeks to get used to eating three square meals per day. Over this time, we also worked on food quality and upping her fat and lowering her carbohydrate consumption. Mary Ann also had low vitamin D, so adding that in along with omega-3 fatty acids and ACV, were keys to her success. Mary Ann did a lot of work at home on her sleep, stress response, and meal timing, but we agreed she would scale way back on the exercise from what she had been doing.

At the one-month mark, Mary Ann began experimenting with fasting, increasing it to 12 hours, and then 16 hours six weeks into the plan. It was critical that she take things low and slow in order to maintain the lifestyle, but Mary Ann was frustrated at the one-month mark. I like to point this out because, although Mary Ann's waist measurements started to drop at six weeks, she really needed to trust me in the interim. Two weeks in, Mary Ann felt mentally clearer, less stressed, and had less pain in her body. She noticed her energy skyrocket and her cravings drop off by four weeks, but still no significant change in her body composition. Why? It takes time to start to see changes if you're significantly insulin resistant. Those insulin levels need to come down, and it's not worth beating them into submission if you want success in the long term. By the 12-week mark, the new lifestyle changes seemed effortless to Mary Ann, and they easily fit into her life, almost as easily as she fit into her pants. She was back into the clothes that she wore after her first pregnancy and was on her way to her pre-pregnancy weight.

What was better still, Mary Ann felt confident in her body and empowered to make decisions about when to eat "off plan." She now knew how foods affected her body; she finally understood how her body worked! Mary Ann said something to me in our latest visit that resonated: the number on the scale had only mattered to her because she felt that was the only feedback she got from her body. She had never been taught to measure her waist, track her energy, or use her cravings and confidence as a guide. Like myself, Mary Ann no longer cared about the number on the scale because she felt at home in her body and in control over the outcome. This is what I want for you as well.

What Is Insulin?

Recall the discussion of digestion as a hormonal process. Food enters the small intestine for absorption. If that food is a carbohydrate, or a sugary food, then it will increase both blood sugar and insulin levels. (Interestingly, protein also increases insulin levels, although it has a minimal effect on glucose [sugar], whereas fat does not have a remarkable effect on either insulin or glucose.) Therefore, when you eat a meal of carbohydrates or protein, your insulin will rise as part of the digestive hormonal response.

As mentioned, insulin is a hormone involved with blood sugar regulation, fat storage, ovulation and reproductive hormones, acne, and skin health. When it comes to hormones they all work on the same principle: a lock and key system. A hormone (the key) binds to receptors (the lock), opening the door to a whole host of processes that allow the hormone to exert its function. When insulin, for instance, is released in response to food intake, it binds to its receptors in our cells and sweeps blood sugar out of the bloodstream into storage.

Insulin Resistance

Normal Fasting
· Able to use fat as fuel
· Normal insulin (keys)
· Normal glucose (balls)

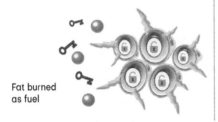

Fat burned as fuel

Normal Response After Eating
· Appropriate insulin glucose response
· Normal insulin
· Normal glucose

Glucose absorbed into cells

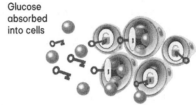

Increased insulin – Fasting
· NOT able to use fat as fuel efficiently
· Increased insulin
· Normal glucose

Fat cells increase in size

Some glucose absorbed into cells

Insulin Resistance after eating
· Inappropriate insulin glucose response
· Increased insulin
· Increased glucose

Glucose not absorbed into cells

Fat cells increase in size

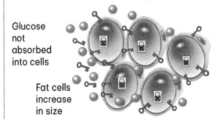

Figure 13. In a normal state, insulin (keys) will bind to the insulin receptors (locks) and allow glucose to leave the blood stream and enter the cells. Insulin and glucose will rise and then fall normally with meals so that your body is able to use fat as fuel overnight and between meals as well. As insulin resistance progresses, fasting insulin increases and the ability to use fat as fuel over-night is diminished. If this pattern continues, glucose and insulin will elevate together in a fed state, meaning your body is still storing fuel and is unable to use fat as fuel efficiently.

When your blood sugar elevates during a meal, your insulin will also increase in order to store that blood sugar in the liver or muscles as glycogen or in our *adipo-cytes* (fat cells) as fat for later use. The body has an order in which all of this storage happens. After glucose is absorbed for immediate use by cells, any left over is first stored in the liver and muscles as glycogen. After these glycogen stores are filled, your fat cells become the storage destination of choice. As you can imagine, these fat stores are an expanding storage site; therefore, your body continually shuttles blood sugar away here to guard against the negative effects of high glucose levels in the bloodstream (these effects include issues with circulation, vision changes, kidney damage, and even infection). So your fat stores are critical to your health.

In order to get fuel out of storage, insulin levels need to be low. When you enter a fasting period, such as going from dinner to breakfast without eating, insulin levels should drop very low, allowing another hormone, glucagon, to trigger the release of glucose from the liver glycogen stores. During this time, you also need proper levels of cortisol, epinephrine, and norepinephrine to help to liberate sugar stores. You will notice there are many redundant systems in the body to protect important functions. Glucose is critical to cellular function; in fact, glucose is needed by every cell in the body and is the preferred source of fuel for the brain. Anticipating that humans will go through periods of fasting, or even famine, the body has multiple levels of glucose storage to draw from. Kind of like squirrels storing away nuts for the winter, your body stores away glucose in the form of glycogen in the liver and muscles, and fat in our fat cells.

Here's important information: the body taps into liver and muscle glycogen first in times of fasting, not your fat stores. This has a huge impact on weight loss, because if you are not spending time in the fasted state, you will only be drawing from your liver and muscle stores for fuel, which leaves your fat cells quite comfy and plump. If you are eating all day long, snacking between meals, and having that one last snack before bed, your fasting to feeding ratio is way off, no matter how many calories you're eating. We are set up to have at least 12 hours per day in the fasted state, and less than 12 hours per day in the fed state. Otherwise, insulin levels will be high, and so will your body fat percentage. If you want your body to be in fat-burning mode, then proper control of satiety hormones (PYY, CCK, incretins) and low insulin levels along with proper adrenal hormone support are critical.

Table 7. Hormonal environment in the fed and fasted state

Hormones of the Fed State (aka Storage Mode)	Hormones of the Fasted State (aka Burning Mode)
High insulin levels	Low insulin levels
CKK elevates	Glucagon rises
PYY elevates	Epinephrine, Norepinephrine increase
GLP-1/GIP elevates	Cortisol may increase

Fuel Store Rank

NO Fat Burning

Fat stored in your cells is like food in the freezer. Food in the freezer needs to be thawed, so it's not immediately accessible.

Glycogen is like food in the fridge. It's available immediately!

When insulin is high this increases glycogen storage and further inhibits fat burning.

↑Insulin
Sugar burning

Body Fat

Glycogen

Fuel Store Rank

Fat burning

When you fast, it's as though your fridge is empty and you start to access the food in the freezer – the fat.

↓Insulin
NO Sugar Burning

Body Fat

Glycogen

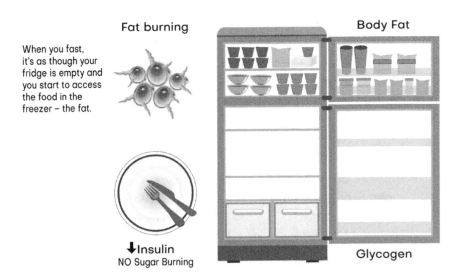

Figure 14. Glycogen stored in the liver and muscles acts as the fridge form of glucose storage. Food stored in the fridge is easy to use. In contrast, energy stored in the fat cells is analogous to food stored in the freezer. Your body

will generally first use the fuel in the fridge because it takes a while to thaw the frozen fuel. Therefore, if your insulin is high and you have glycogen in the muscles and liver, your body will use those stores. If you are in a fasted state, and the fridge is empty, your body will tap into the fat stores to burn as fuel.

Glucose, Glucagon, and Glycogen
Terminology can get confusing. When discussing the metabolic system, there are three main G's to know and differentiate. *Glucose*, also known as sugar, is what we measure in the blood and what your brain and other organs use as fuel. *Glucagon* is kind of like the anti-insulin. When your blood glucose begins to drop, the pancreas releases the hormone glucagon, which works to increase blood glucose by stimulating the breakdown of glycogen in the liver. *Glycogen* is the storage form of glucose in the liver.

How Insulin Changes Throughout the Day

Proper insulin function prevents diabetes, so let's not hate the player, or the game for that matter! Many of us come from a place of disdain for our bodies and for food, but we need to flip that paradigm on its head so that we do not also develop disdain for our hormones, especially when they are just trying to do their jobs. Remember, there is such thing as a healthy insulin response.

When you wake in the morning, your glucose and insulin levels should be low. This is, of course, dependent on having fasted overnight for at least 12 hours. You should have spent the night burning glycogen and fat as your fuel and wake feeling ready for the day after a period of metabolic hormone reset. Upon eating your first meal, your insulin levels will increase slowly, peaking between 30 and 60 minutes after your meal. Throughout this period your glucose is kept under control, and then insulin and glucose levels should decrease back to baseline within three to four hours of your meal.

When this system works properly, your body should be able to seamlessly move from using your meal to fuel your energy to using your energy stores (fat and glycogen) for energy. There should be no shakiness, no anxiety, no feeling of overwhelm, and no drive to devour the cookie jar at the office. This was not the case for me back in the day!

When I was younger, my mother carried granola bars with her everywhere. I would go from hungry-ish one minute to hangry the next. I had crazy blood sugar swings. I had brain fog, food-related anxiety, and I was unable to go more than four hours without having a meal or snack. All this while still having 80–100 lbs of extra fat on my body, weight that I would have loved to be able to use up. I wish I could speak to my previous self and tell her that her "healthy" diet was completely aggravating her symptoms, working against her goals, and preventing her from using that fat as fuel. I wish I could tell her what I am able to share with you in this book!

When Insulin Signalling Goes Wrong

Hands down the number one questions that I get is, "Why can my friend eat all the sugar she wants, and if I so much as look at a bagel I gain 5 lbs?" Of course, the answer is complex, involving genetics, inflammation levels, whatever else your friend ate that day, but, it also has a lot to do with how *your* body releases and responds to insulin. Something about your insulin response is different than that of your friend's. Something has gone wrong.

Although insulin has long been associated with obesity, a normal insulin response does not result in obesity; it just results in a healthy stable blood sugar level and seamless transition between meals. As your body moves away from the healthy insulin response, there's a creeping up in insulin levels, for years if not decades, before it's detected in routine physical blood work. What you will see initially is an elevated or prolonged insulin response to a meal, resulting in more insulin exposure and, therefore, more fat storage and less fat burning. This response continues as the cells become more and more insulin resistant, the key just not fitting in the lock effectively. When this continues for a long time we see more inflammation, more nutrient overload and more cortisol demands. The result, you need more insulin for the lock to open and insulin sticks around longer to keep glucose under control. You will also start to see an elevation in fasting insulin, meaning you aren't even in fat-burning mode overnight (see fig. 13). At this point the trouble has really set in, and the response is precipitous fat gain.

This process occurs even before you see changes in fasting glucose, before pre-diabetes, and long before type 2 diabetes develops. This is the period of time when you are overweight, feel awful, depend on sugar for fuel, have cravings, bad skin, possibly even fertility issues, yet, somehow, you are still "normal" and there's nothing wrong with you on a typical blood panel ordered by a primary care medical doctor. This is where you need to look further and take action.

There are countless theories about why, or how, the body becomes insulin resistant. A few of them include:

- Genetics (although your genes are not your destiny)
- Nutrition overload and oxidative stress
- Chronically elevated insulin levels
- Fructose consumption

- Elevated levels of lipopolysaccharide (LPS) and gut inflammation (think metabolic endotoxemia)

Due to the fact that the *why* is still a bit of a guessing game, I think it's more important to focus on lowering your insulin stimulation, supporting receptors, and encouraging a proper cycle of fed and fasting states. As I update this book in the future, I may have more information about the why. For now, let's focus on the hundreds of pounds lost and the energy and body confidence gained on the Finally Lose It Program, and get you the success you crave, just like Mary Ann.

Leptin Resistance and the Fat Stat

Research shows that leptin, discussed in **chapter 3**, and insulin resistance go hand in hand. Elevated levels of insulin actually induce leptin resistance. As mentioned in **chapter 4**, leptin is a hormone created by your fat cells and tells your body just how much energy you have stored. The more fat you have, the more leptin is released. Leptin messages your brain, "Oh hey, you have plenty of stores. Maybe you should stop eating, increase the metabolism, and move around a bit more."

In some circles the leptin-insulin relationship is called the "fat stat" because it functions to keep our weight within a certain range. Just like a thermostat regulating heat in a home, your body decides how much fat it wants and will defend that. When leptin is working well, it works **with** us.

Research has been done on a very rare genetic condition in which people do not synthesize any leptin. These people experience continual ravenous hunger, a slower metabolism, and no inherent drive to move. In these cases, injecting leptin into the system normalized their appetite, increased their metabolism, and normalized their weight. Here's where the research waters get muddied: obese people without a genetic leptin deficiency were found to have elevated levels of leptin. When they were injected with even more leptin on a trial basis, nothing happened. What is happening here?

Well, just as with insulin, it's not all about the amount of hormone circulating. Yes, enough insulin is important, but too much is not protective or helpful. The same principle applies with leptin: too much can actually lead to leptin resistance. The brain stops listening to the signals from your fat cells. In this situation, your fat stat thinks you are lean, even though you've got plenty of fat that you would love your body to use as fuel. Your metabolism slows, your energy and basal movement levels tank, and you feel like you are trudging your way through the day on willpower because your appetite is out of control. It's the perfect storm for weight loss resistance, and although there's nothing abnormal on your blood work panel, you know there must be something wrong.

Insulin Resistance Quiz

1) What is your waist measurement?
   a. Waist > 35 inches
   a. Small frame and waist > 32 inches
   b. Waist < 35/32 inches

2) Do you gain weight predominantly on your abdomen and trunk?
   a. Yes
   b. No

3) Do you crave sweets and sugar?
   a. Yes
   b. No

4) Do you struggle with weight loss? Or gain weight easily?
   a. Yes
   b. No

5) Do you crave carbohydrates, rice, bread, or pasta?
   a. Yes
   b. No

6) Do you struggle to limit food at meals, or tend to binge eat?
   a. Yes
   b. No

7) Do you have a family history of diabetes, or have you had gestational diabetes?
   a. Yes
   b. No

8) Do you, or others in your family, have non-alcoholic fatty liver (NAFLD)?
   a. Yes
   b. No

9) Do you have polycystic ovarian syndrome (PCOS)?
   a. Yes
   b. No

10) Do you have adult acne?
    a. Yes
    b. No

11) Do you have patches of skin on your neck, armpit, groin, and other creases

that are dark and velvety? (aka acanthosis nigricans)

    a.   Yes

    b.   No

12) Do you tend to get skin tags?

    a.   Yes

    b.   No

13) Do you struggle to keep your blood sugar stable? Do you ever feel hangry, shaky, dizzy, or unwell if you go too long without eating?

    a.   Yes

    b.   No

If you answered yes (or chose A) in more than eight of those questions, you have some work to do. Don't be discouraged or overwhelmed if you are checking yes to every quiz in this book. It's no surprise that your body isn't working properly. If it were, you would not need to read this. I have laid out a 30-day plan for you to take the information from each of these chapters and implement it in a manageable way. You can do it!

"REALISTICALLY, YOU PROBABLY SPEND THE MAJORITY OF YOUR WAKING HOURS EATING, DRINKING, OR THINKING ABOUT FOOD; THEREFORE, WHY WOULD YOU TAKE THE RESULTS OF A FASTING TEST AND INTERPRET HEALTH BASED ON THAT?"

Testing for Insulin Resistance

There are many lab tests that your medical doctor will run to investigate the health of your blood sugar response. The most common ones are fasting blood glucose and the hemoglobin A1c (HbA1c). These tests, although valuable to diagnose diabetes, do not tell you much about your fat loss potential.

Fasting blood glucose is exactly what it sounds like. It's a measurement of how much sugar is in your bloodstream after you have not eaten for a 12-hour period. The test can tell you if you are diabetic, but it will not tell you how much insulin is required to shuttle that glucose away. Similarly, HbA1c is a marker of the average blood sugar level over the course of three months. Although being within the normal range of these markers is good, it definitely does not mean that you're in a healthy fat-burning state.

Fasting insulin can be a valuable marker in people with frank hyperinsulinemia (high insulin release) or insulin resistance. As discussed above, the initial response of insulin resistance is not always one of elevated fasting insulin, but instead it can be elevated insulin following a meal. So again, this test is helpful, but it doesn't tell you the whole story about your insulin and glucose response.

The New Paradigm of Testing for Fat Loss

Enter the two-hour insulin and glucose response test. This test is the best tool we currently have to assess metabolic hormones and how they respond in a fed state. Realistically, you probably spend the majority of your waking hours eating, drinking, or thinking about food; therefore, why would you take the results of a fasting test and interpret health based on that? Doesn't make sense, does it?

One particular researcher, Dr. Joseph Kraft, used this logic to change the game when it comes to understanding the patterns of hyperinsulinemia and insulin resistance, and how to test for them. He tested thousands of people, looking at how they responded to glucose over a two-hour period. He found that in obese people there is an elevation in insulin. This elevation marks the progression toward blood sugar dysregulation and diabetes. The moral of the story is that we need to be testing and treating insulin resistance long before your conventional lab work looks "abnormal."

Before you have a complete panic attack, however, let's make something crystal clear: insulin resistance is not a destination or a one-way track to diabetes! It's reversible at every stage and is 100% possible to change when you are empowered with the right information. With diet, lifestyle, the recommendations laid out in this book, and the 30-day-kick start plan in the final section, you can (and will, if I have anything to say about it) reverse insulin resistance, get into fat-burning mode, overcome your weight loss plateaus, and feel at your best in your body.

What Is a Normal Insulin Response?

A "normal" test for insulin and glucose includes a rise in insulin and glucose that peaks at 30 minutes after consuming a very sugary standardized drink. Glucose levels should be less than 7 mmol/L (125 mg/dL) and insulin levels around 500 pmol/L (72 units/mL) at this time. After two hours, glucose levels should be between 5 and

6 mmol/L (90-108 mg/dL). Insulin levels should also steadily fall to reach an insulin level no higher than 220 pmol/L after two hours (<32 units/mL). (See appendix A for a summary of this data and unit conversions.) However, these values are rarely the case. Estimates suggest that only 20% of the population is truly normo-responsive to a glucose load. This has held true of what I have seen in my clinical practice, and also when I first tested myself. There are endless ways this response can go awry, and it will be different in each of you. Having seen many of these in my own patients, and in working with my colleague who introduced me to this test, Dr. Fiona McCulloch (who does amazing work with PCOS), we have found this test incredibly valuable as we can customize the diet, lifestyle, and supplement approaches based on the results.

Below is a simplified version of the insulin responses as insulin resistance progresses. These responses are all prior to type 2 diabetes onset. Have a look at the advanced insulin resistance (IR). If higher insulin leads to more difficulty losing weight, imagine how difficult it will be as the levels continue to climb.

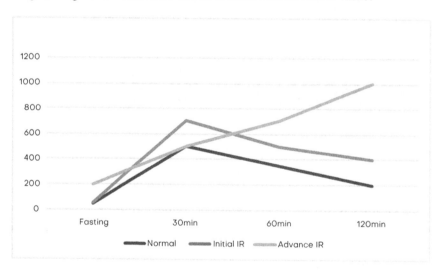

Figure 15. Dr. Joseph Kraft depicted in his research patterns of insulin resistance. In a normal case, insulin is low fasting, rising to its highest by 30 minutes and then slowly falling to appropriate levels by 120 minutes after the glucose is consumed. As insulin resistance progresses, the insulin response is higher after meals, and although it falls by 120 minutes, it does not drop down to baseline. In the third state, advanced insulin resistance, insulin levels start high and continue to rise 120 minutes after meals. This is a state of perpetual storage mode, inflammation, and insulin resistance.

How Foods Affect Normal Insulin Production

Remember when I mentioned, in the introduction, that I went on a "no whites" diet? It was the first time that I truly felt the powerful effects of food on my body. At that time, I had no idea how it worked, all I knew was that it did—for a while. Despite my initial success, losing 50 lbs, I continued to hit plateaus. I had been indoctrinated to believe that low fat was the way to go, and a no whites diet is by definition a lower carb diet, which left me hungry a lot of the time and also eating a lot of protein. At the time, I had no clue; the glycemic index told me that protein was a great choice for my glucose control, but I had a hunch that this wasn't the whole story. This was when I put my research skills to work.

"THIS WAS THE FIRST TIME THAT THE LITERATURE HAD SUPPORTED MY BELIEF THAT EVERY BITE OF FOOD IS A HORMONAL EXPERIENCE."

Glycemic Index versus Food Insulin Demand

The glycemic index is a measurement of how much a food increases blood sugar. This system, although helpful, is incomplete because we do not gain weight due to blood sugar levels. We gain weight because of insulin. If you're really interested in overcoming weight loss resistance, you need to be more concerned with how much insulin your pancreas releases in response to a food, not your glucose response. And luckily, this research has been done.

The moment that I began to dig into the research on food insulin demand (FID) I knew that I had the potential to change for the better the way weight loss is approached. This was the first time the literature had supported my belief that every bite of food is a *hormonal* experience. It also explained why fad diets that overly restrict fat or focus too heavily on carbs and protein fail in the long term. In the FID research study, researchers measured how much insulin is released in response to consumption of specific foods. This study further confirmed the theories that carbohydrates increase insulin. It also added to the picture that milk has an unusually significant effect on insulin, and the combination of fat and carbohydrates (such as a croissant or pizza) spikes the insulin response even higher than carbs on their own.[85,86] This may not surprise a lot of you, as we know that deep-fried foods, chips, chocolate, pizza, etc., are not exactly friendly to the waistline. As mentioned, fat is a macronutrient that eaten alone does *not* increase insulin. Yes, fat in the form of healthy fats does not make us fat when eaten in a healthy context. Indeed, fat is critical to our reproductive hormone balance, to our brain health, and to our cellular health. Goodbye to the theory carried on for generations that fat is simply bad!

I will go so far as to say that the low-fat fads have contributed to the current obesity epidemic. I know, it seems a grandiose statement, but low-fat diets are by definition high in carbohydrates. When you read a food package, you can see it for yourself. Food manufacturers take out the fat—the fat that keeps your blood sugar stable and that keeps you feeling full and satisfied—and they add sugar to ensure the food still tastes good. This is bad news for all of us who have insulin signalling issues, which I would argue is the majority of the population.

What about the macronutrient protein on the insulin index? As mentioned, protein does not have a significant effect on the blood sugar response, and a high-protein diet has been touted for years as a weight loss tactic. However, it proves to be another failed tactic because protein increases insulin in a manner similar to some carbohydrates. One of the theories as to why protein stimulates insulin suggests that it actually has nothing to do with fat loss or gain. In a healthy body, insulin also has a function to help shuttle amino acids (small pieces that make up protein) into the muscles; therefore, consumption of protein supports muscle development. But if you are insulin resistant or hyperinsulinemic, adding more insulin to an already overflowing bucket results in issues with fat gain. In this situation, knowing what your insulin levels are at fasting and how your body responds to carbohydrates is a game changer. This information helps to ensure you get enough protein, but not too much, and enough carbohydrates, but not too many. In other words, blood work helps to find the sweet spot for resetting your insulin and your fat stat. This is exactly how the diet plan is set up in **chapter 9**.

Fructose: Is All Sugar the Same?

Fructose, sucrose, glucose, essentially anything ending in –*ose*, represent different carbohydrate sugars. Is sugar just sugar though? The answer is no. All sugars have a different effect on insulin levels and insulin resistance in the body. Out of all of these varieties, it's important to consider fructose. For decades scientists have been raising the "maybe not a good idea" flag regarding the ubiquitous use of high-fructose corn syrup and similar high-fructose sweeteners. The reason for this? Diets high in fructose have been shown to decrease insulin signalling and increase insulin levels compared to its glucose counterpart.[87,88] This is a significant issue that undoubtedly contributes to the growth of waistlines. When I talk about foods high in fructose I am not referencing fruit of any sort. We have no reason to believe that fruit in moderation is an issue. What I am talking about is soda/pop, other sweetened drinks, candy, and processed foods sweetened with fructose. Avoid this ingredient where possible.

Take Action
Sugar comes in many guises in processed foods. Common names for sugar on labels include: corn sweetener, corn syrup, dextrose, fructose, fruit juice concentrates, glucose, high-fructose corn syrup, invert sugar, lactose, maltose, malt syrup, raw sugar, sucrose, sugar syrup, cane crystals, cane sugar, crystalline fructose, evaporated cane juice, corn syrup solids, and malt syrup. Please read the labels.

"WHAT I ASK YOU TO RECOGNIZE IS THAT WHAT YOU'VE BEEN DOING HAS NOT WORKED FOR YOU, AND YOU STILL HAVE QUESTIONS. OTHERWISE, YOU WOULDN'T BE HERE, READING THIS BOOK. SO LET'S OPTIMIZE THE OPPORTUNITY FOR A NEW PATH."

Do We Need to Care about Calories?

Newsflash: you should be able to eat between 2,000 and 3,000 calories per day and lose weight. When your hormones are in balance and you are eating a low-carb, moderate protein, moderate fat diet, you can live in an optimal space of health eating to your satisfaction and lose weight. I don't mind telling you that this blew my understanding that calories were critical out of the water. Don't get me wrong, calories matter to some extent, as does how well your thyroid is working (see appendix A) and how insulin resistant you are, but calories are by no means the be-all and end-all. You already know that though, because if you are anything like me, you've tried (and been surrounded by others) eating 1,000 calories per day of carbohydrates and still not losing weight. This is where understanding how macronutrients (fat, carbs, and protein) affect your body is critical. Again, you cannot eat 10,000 calories per day and expect to have a healthy body or metabolic response—but fat loss is much more about hormones when we are talking about weight loss resistance.

I understand that I'm asking a lot of you: I'm asking you to change your perception and to recognize that you have been brainwashed by the industry to eat and live in a way that we now know makes people feel fat, sick, and a little crazy. What I ask you to recognize is that what you've been doing has not worked for you, and you still have questions. Otherwise, you wouldn't be here, reading this book. So let's optimize the opportunity for a new path. Tinker with your health according to the guidelines I set out in this book to discover what your body is trying to tell you and what your body is capable of.

Meal Timing and Insulin Response

I discuss meal timing in the context of circadian rhythm in **chapter 2**. You'll recall that your meals should be consumed during daylight hours, which is when your digestive enzymes and hormones are primed and waiting to receive food. Eating late at night just doesn't fly. Even people with healthy metabolism who eat during the circadian night will see results in elevated glucose and insulin levels that are on par with someone with diabetes. But what about meals during the day? Should you eat three meals, six meals? This is where we need to consider insulin.

"MEAL TIMING AND LEAVING TIME BETWEEN MEALS TO ALLOW YOUR METABOLIC HORMONES TO RESET IS GOING TO BE CRITICAL TO YOUR JOURNEY. IF YOU CURRENTLY EAT FIVE MEALS PER DAY OR THREE

MEALS AND TWO SNACKS, OR WORSE, IF YOU GRAZE THROUGHOUT THE DAY AND DON'T EAT PROPER MEALS AT ALL, THERE IS ROOM FOR IMPROVEMENT."

As I am my own personal experiment, I'm constantly playing around with different eating styles, exercises, routines, and personal development strategies. One particular time I was experimenting with an "if it fits my macros"–style bodybuilding diet and workout plan. I was at the gym every day lifting weights, sprinting, and kicking my own butt. I was also eating five to six small meals a day. They were healthy meals too: smoothies, high protein, moderate fat, and moderate to high carb. I followed the equation to a tee, and guess what? I gained weight! I am sure that you have felt this frustration a time or two, when you are busting your butt, eating "clean," and doing everything you are told to do and more. I was at the point where I wanted to give up! Instead, I did what I always do when I'm in investigator mode: I dove into the research to find an answer.

At this point, I knew about insulin and my tendency toward insulin resistance. But from everything I had read, a high-carb diet was the issue and burst-type training, along with weight training, was necessary to reverse that insulin resistance. I thought I would be fine, and of course it looked like everyone else was changing their bodies on this plan. (See, even I fall for these fads!) As I dug deeper and deeper into the research, I started to see commentaries that brought into question this way of eating. I put this together with the Kraft research, discussed above, and it all clicked.

Insulin response without Snacking

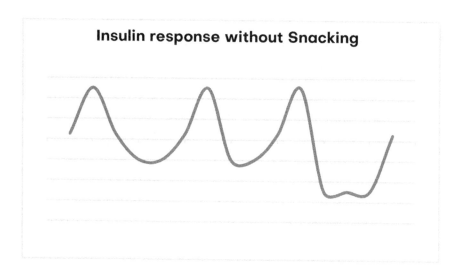

Figure 16. Insulin levels should rise with three meals per day and drop between meals and overnight, allowing a balanced fed versus fasting state.

When you are insulin resistant, or even hypersensitive to insulin, eating five meals per day or snacking throughout the day is going to drive your body into fat storage mode. Remember that insulin has a very important role in taking blood sugar out of your bloodstream after your meal and shuttling it into storage. Therefore, with every meal insulin needs time to rise and fall (see fig. 16). When this system is working well, insulin and glucose levels should be down to fasting levels by three to four hours after your meals. When insulin remains high though, and the body is in fat storage mode, your ability to use fat as fuel is reduced, leading to that "tire" of resistant belly fat and persistent cravings and desire for food. So if your insulin levels haven't come back down to a point where you are using fat before you eat your next meal or snack, the effects are compounding and insulin will rise again. Do you see why I was gaining fat during my multiple small meals a day plan? I was keeping myself in storage mode. Essentially, I busted the one diet for everyone myth!

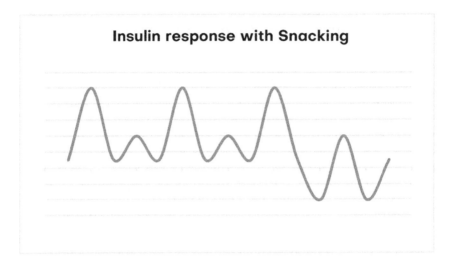

Insulin response with Snacking

Figure 17. If you hope to lose weight, you need to use your "freezer" fat stores as fuel and give your body time to use up all the fuel in the "fridge." Constant snacking raises insulin, essentially refilling the fridge. In addition, snacking can contribute to poor blood sugar control throughout the night, resulting in poor sleep and nighttime awakening.

Meal timing and leaving time between meals to allow your metabolic hormones to reset is going to be critical to your journey. If you currently eat five meals per day or three meals and two snacks, or worse, if you graze throughout the day and don't eat proper meals at all, there is room for improvement. The first step is going to be confining your meals to three 30-minute to 60-minute eating windows. This allows your insulin levels to look like those represented in fig. 16, rising with each meal and falling between meals. We also want to see at a minimum a 10-hour fasting window from the last bite of food you take at night to the first bite of food you take in the morning.

If you are already limiting your eating window to three 1-hour windows, we have more space to play. My ideal world includes extending the fasting window overnight to 12 hours, or even 16 hours as your body becomes more fat-adapted. This is where the magic happens.

Fasting: What Now?
I have to admit, I was opposed to fasting for a long time. My resistance was purely a reflection of not trusting my body, not pushing my boundaries, and not knowing the research. Now, having seen the results for myself and in countless patients, I see the utility of intermittent fasting to overcome weight loss resistance and to

help improve insulin sensitivity. Going long periods without food (water, tea, and black coffee are OK) can allow your insulin levels to drop, your body to use fat as fuel, your leptin signals to begin to reset, and it gets to some of the root causes of insulin resistance, which are related to overnutrition in the cells and cellular oxidative stress. Fasting also has the benefit of lowering inflammation by supporting the immune system. All great things!

Please note, if you take medication for diabetes, cardiovascular disease, or other conditions, don't go beyond a 12-hour overnight fast or change your diet timing drastically without medical supervision. You should also not begin fasting if you are stressed to the max. Fasting is a stress to the body, and just as blood sugar swings are a huge stress to the body, it can work against you to increase cortisol, call on norepinephrine and epinephrine, and alter insulin signalling. If you do not listen to your body, and if you try to push a system that's broken, you just won't get the results you want. If you are burnt out, work on correcting that first. Support your insulin signalling by fasting 12 hours overnight and try to limit snacks when you can. But if you feel like the effort is exhausting and you need to chug coffee or tea to make it from breakfast to lunch, then have a snack, okay?

Fasting is like a muscle, and just as you wouldn't walk into the gym for the first time and try to lift 500 lbs, you shouldn't jump into fasting from eating five meals per day. I often recommend starting with increasing your fasting window by 30 minutes at a time. For example, if you are only fasting eight hours overnight right now, then increase that to eight and a half hours for the next three to four days, then to nine hours, then nine and a half hours, and so forth. When you get to a 12-hour fasting window, hang there for a bit and see how you feel, all while starting to cut out snacks. If you are feeling good, then work toward the goal of a 16-hour fast two to three times per week, moving slowly. All the while checking in with yourself, making sure that you are feeling energized, not exhausted and brain foggy, on fasting days.

Many of my patients' eyes glaze over when I mention fasting. One particular patient, Melanie, is a great example of the power of a personalized diet that includes fasting. She was opposed to any diet changes or to changing her fasting window. Essentially, she was resistant to challenging her boundaries or leaving her comfort zone. Rightly so. Melanie was thirty years old and felt as though she had spent the better part of her life restricting herself, trying to lose the extra 50–70 lbs that would fluctuate on and off her waistline and hips. Melanie was eating the typical points-counting diet, high carb, low fat, moderate to low protein, with tons of snacks and no focus on satiety or nutrient density. It was the only thing that worked for her in the past. To which we had a good laugh when I pointed out, if it was working so well why was she in my office? I set out a 30-day plan to support her through the changes I wanted to see, similar to what I have set out in this book. I gave her all the support that I could and all the education that I felt she needed. We chatted about mindset, challenging boundaries, and she was off to the races. After eight weeks Melanie hadn't come back, so I reached out to see how she was doing, thinking we were going to have to start from scratch. To my surprise, the reason Melanie hadn't returned was that she had lost two dress sizes, lost her cravings, bloating, and fluid retention, and gained her life back. The thing to remember here is that what we eat is incredibly powerful, and so, too, is what (and when) we don't eat.

"IF YOU ARE STILL UNDER THE IMPRESSION THAT YOU CAN OUTRUN A POOR DIET AND THAT THE AMOUNT OF CALORIES YOU BURN ON THE TREADMILL IS IMPERATIVE TO YOUR SUCCESS IN WEIGHT LOSS, THEN I HAVE NEWS FOR YOU."

Exercise: You Can't Outrun a Poor Diet

Exercise is just not what it's cracked up to be when it comes to weight loss. In fact, I'm on a mission to completely change how people think about exercise! If you are still under the impression that you can outrun a poor diet and that the amount of calories you burn on the treadmill is imperative to your success in weight loss, then I have news for you. The reality is that you cannot outrun a pizza, nor can you work off a night of sugary alcohol drinks. It's also true that you cannot burn 200 calories running your little heart out and then "earn" an extra 200 calories from your diet. Why am I talking about exercise then? Well, exercise does have a significant impact on your weight loss goals, but not for the reason you might believe. It is actually how exercise affects your *hormones* that makes the biggest difference.

When it comes to insulin resistance–and changing the hormonal environment to foster weight loss–we want to see our muscles working. Long-distance cardio just won't cut it (and might actually cause you to gain weight). True story. I have had a number of patients training for a half, or full, marathon and mysteriously gain weight. When you're running long distances, your body is calling on cortisol to help fuel your run. Therefore, if you are already in stressed out, cortisol over-drive mode, this can make insulin resistance worse. We need to get most women away from long-distance cardio and into burst exercise and resistance training. This includes weight training like push-ups, squats, lunges, and burpees.

I am no personal trainer, but what I do know is that the research supports the benefits of high-intensity interval training (HIIT) and resistance training.[89,90] Whether you watch workout videos, go to a boot camp, or get a personal trainer is up to you. But if you want to break the cycle of insulin resistance and leptin resistance, you need to get your butt working (literally!). Aim for resistance training two to three times per week at a minimum. When it comes to HIIT, these workouts are generally five to 15 minutes and have been shown to provide the same, or more, benefits as your 60-minute gym outings.[91] The effects of HIIT on your metabolism also last significantly longer than continuous low-intensity exercise. Studies have shown that even 24 hours later your glucose control can still be positively affected.[92] The bonus is that everyone has five to 15 minutes in their day—so no excuses!

Take Action

Movement and exercise are two different things. Movement is critical for your whole health. I hope you understand that sitting is the new smoking! You should be aiming to get in between 8,000 and 10,000 steps per day for general health. Walking, especially in nature, is also one of my favourite forms of movement, as it can lower cortisol. So make sure you are incorporating walking into your daily life, above and beyond exercise, at least two to three times per week.

Supplements

I will not be recommending a wide assortment of supplements in this chapter because, first, the diet and lifestyle changes I discussed are so powerful, and second, because all the supplements and steps I've recommended thus far are contributing to improving your insulin sensitivity and weight loss goals. There are a few very powerful supplements to consider though, my favourites being vitamin D, omega-3 fatty acids, and ACV.

Note: You do not need everything on the supplement list accruing in this book. Check in at each chapter and choose only the supplements that feel right to you or that have been selected specifically for you by your healthcare professional.

Vitamin D

Vitamin D is the "sunshine hormone." The pathway to make vitamin D in the body includes the sun shining on your skin, though this is just the first step. When you are exposed to sun, 7-dehydrocholesterol turns into pre-vitamin D3 and then to vitamin D3. Vitamin D3 then has to be taken to the liver to be turned into 25-OH vitamin D3 and then to the kidney to be turned into 1,25-OH² vitamin D3, which is the most active form of vitamin D. These are the forms we refer to when we reference vitamin D.[93]

If you're up here in the Northern Hemisphere like me, it's incredibly difficult to make vitamin D from the sun, and most people need to take supplements to get their vitamin D to adequate levels. Those rumours that 20 minutes of sun exposure are enough to make adequate vitamin D only applies if you're exposing the majority of your body, not wearing sunscreen, and it's between April and October. I don't know about you, but I am not often chilling in the nude in my yard during peak sun hours in *any* month, so I test my levels and supplement appropriately!

Vitamin D has innumerable functions in the body. Its importance truly cannot be underestimated. It is a master regulator of our immune system, controlling autoimmune disease and inflammation levels. It is also related to our hormonal balance, as vitamin D is itself a fat soluble hormone and is a signalling molecule in the body. There's also extensive research on the role of vitamin D in insulin resistance, weight loss resistance, diabetes, and metabolic syndrome. If you do not have sufficient levels of vitamin D, whether you are overweight or not, your body is still metabolically unhealthy. You are at increased risk of obesity, inflammation, cholesterol issues, and insulin resistance when your vitamin D levels are suboptimal.[93,94] This is why supplementing based on lab testing is important. If you have enough of the sunshine hormone, then taking more will not help you. Alternatively, if you are low, you need to get supplementing if you want a body that's insulin sensitive and burning fat. Supplementing at adequate levels for your deficiency status has also been shown to be important. For example, supplementing 400 IU in a deficient adult had no positive effect on insulin resistance or weight, whereas 4,000 IU or more had a significant benefit in many studies.[93]

Take Action

Vitamin D is fat soluble, so it should be taken with a meal containing fat, and ideally should be supplemented in a fat matrix—oil or emulsified drop for best absorption. Unlike some of the B vitamins, vitamin D is not simply peed out of your body when you take in excess; therefore, it's important to know your levels before your start supplementing anything over 1,000 IU per day. With any good thing, too much can lead to toxic levels, which are harmful, just like low levels.

Omega-3 Fatty Acids

As we saw in **chapter 5**, omega-3 fatty acids can be incredibly supportive in reducing inflammation, lowering metabolic endotoxemia, and supporting weight loss. Other studies support a direct effect of omega-3 fatty acids on insulin signalling, potentially because they improve the health of the fatty cell membrane, where the insulin receptors live. Research suggests that women benefit from omega-3 fatty acids to a greater degree than men when it comes to insulin resistance and weight loss. Additionally, remember that you want a high EPA fish oil, ideally with at least 1,500 mg of EPA per serving.[95] This is also going to be most beneficial in people who experience elevated levels of inflammation either symptomatically or on blood testing. For a list of recommended blood tests see appendix A.

Ensure that you take your omega-3 fatty acids with food. This helps to prevent the fishy burp back and increases absorption.

"YOU HAVE LIKELY NOT COME AT DIET AND LIFESTYLE CHANGES FROM A PLACE OF SELF-LOVE, SUPPORT, AND EVIDENCE-BASED SYSTEMS. YOU PROBABLY HAVE NOT WORKED ON YOUR BELIEFS ABOUT BEING TOO BUSY, ABOUT YOUR CAPACITY TO BE HEALTHY, BEAUTIFUL, AND SUCCESSFUL AT EVERY SIZE, AND YOU PROBABLY HAVE NOT CHALLENGED YOUR BELIEFS ABOUT YOUR DESERVINGNESS. YOU ARE HERE THOUGH, WHICH MEANS THAT YOU ARE READY."

Apple Cider Vinegar

Apple cider vinegar can decrease insulin levels. The skeptic in me did not believe this when I heard it. So of course, I dug into the research, and turns out it's true.

Research suggests that 20 g of ACV can increase your insulin sensitivity 19–34%, lowering both the insulin and glucose response to a high-carbohydrate meal.[96] Another study showed improvements in insulin and glucose levels with the addition of 2 Tbsp. of ACV before meals.[97] Additionally, it has been shown to improve fasting glucose levels when taken at night.[98] These results have been repeated in numerous studies in both humans and animals, so that was enough to catch my attention.

Take Action
Go low and slow with your addition of ACV. Start with 1–2 tsp. in a bit of water 15 minutes before your meals. If you feel a burning in your stomach or esophagus, try taking it with a meal. If that still doesn't work, then skip this one. If you are feeling great, increase to 1 Tbsp.

More than a Low-Carb Diet

Right about now, I bet your inner resistance is sabotaging you, telling you that you're not going to succeed, that you've tried a low-carb diet and it didn't work, telling you that you're destined to be overweight forever, and that you may as well devour the chocolate because this plan won't be worth your time. Before that thinking runs away with you, allow me to dispel some myths. You have likely not come at diet and lifestyle changes from a place of self-love, support, and evidence-based systems. You probably have not worked on your beliefs about being too busy, about your capacity to be healthy, beautiful, and successful at every size, and you probably have not challenged your beliefs about your deservingness. You are here though, which means that you *are* ready. And girl, we are going to get you to the finish line! We will be the examples for those women who haven't made it this far yet, and we're going to find them and help them along that path when they are ready. For now though, let's revisit why your past diet, whatever the type, did not work so that you can feel confident going into this one.

I am not advocating a simple low-carb diet here. And I don't think that Atkins is going to change the world for all of us insulin resistant folks. As I mentioned, I have tried it. Yes, it gets you started, but the plateau on a high-protein, nutrient-poor, snack-heavy diet is a real issue! Not to mention that if you have a gut infection, you're taking that high-fat diet and sweeping inflammation into your body. The same is true of many other diets that are targeted to the general population. They are helpful to some, but they do not address the specific issues that we have, all of us lovely ladies who do all the "right things" and still carry extra weight. We need something different. We need something specific. We need this system to address insulin resistance, inflammation, stress, gut issues, the circadian rhythm, and quality sleep. To tackle all of this, we also need to support our mindset, because it takes a freaking toll putting yourself into something and feeling like a failure at the end, doesn't it?

The Finally Lose It Insulin Review

- Insulin is a hormone that plays a critical function in the body: to take sugar from the bloodstream and put it into storage so your body can access that fuel in times of starvation. The problem is, we rarely fast or go without eating, never mind starve.
- Insulin resistance begins with an elevated insulin response to meals, then an elevated baseline level of insulin, and during this process your response to insulin decreases. At that point your body starts to make more and more of this fat storage hormone while your glucose creeps up, which aggravates the whole process.
- Insulin resistance impacts your weight loss by preventing you from using the fat in your body as fuel. This changes your fat stat, leading your brain to think you're lean, so your appetite, your metabolism, and your hormones change to protect you from losing more weight.
- It's time for a diet low in carbs, rich in nutrients, polyphenols, and fibre, that's satiating and has low insulin demand.
- Ensure your protein consumption does not exceed your needs.
- Fasting windows and reducing snacks are imperative to a healthy metabolism and fat stat. If you want to use fat as fuel, give your body a few extra hours without food to help encourage it to break into your fat stores.
- High-intensity exercise is a time and metabolism saver, increasing insulin sensitivity. Exercise can be all about changing your hormones.
- Supplements such as vitamin D, omega-3 FAs, and ACV can support insulin responsiveness.

WHETHER YOU THINK YOU CAN, OR
YOU THINK YOU CAN'T—
YOU'RE RIGHT.

—HENRY FORD

7

GET YOUR HEAD IN THE GAME

You have made promises to yourself that you have not kept, you have felt exhausted, you have given in, you have felt like your body is betraying you, and you have felt overwhelmed by all the diet options. You have tried everything, pretty much, without success, and that feeling of constant failure prevents you from starting again. You don't trust your body anymore and probably feel like everything works against you, while everything seems to work for everyone else, and you just don't get it. But I get you and the scenario you are facing.

That's why this book has a whole chapter devoted to mindset, to getting your mind back in the game. You may read through this book and feel overwhelmed, and that's fair. It is, after all, a compilation of all of the things that I have gone through for decades to lose weight, improve my health, optimize my experience in the world, and feel at home in my body again. I'm going to walk you through this, cheer you on, with this book and the workbook, just like I do with all of my patients. Because like them, I know you can lose 10, 15, 30, 50, or more pounds and feel good in your body! I have seen it in myself, in them; you will succeed too!

I have one specific patient, Monica, who, one year in, just started to unravel. We corrected a lot of the health issues causing her pain, fatigue, and anxiety. We explored all different systems of her body, and she was doing so well. But she still hadn't lost the weight she wanted. We realized that in her case, stress and sleep were still beating on her insulin resistance. We had gone through insulin, when to eat, and what to eat. Then one day she came in, after cancelling a few appointments, and she asked, "What are your thoughts on self-sabotage?" I knew in that moment she was ready for the next phase.

Get Acquainted with Yourself

I always introduce mindset into my patient visits because we *all* need this. You likely have been broken and abused by the diet industry. It has not only taken your money, but parts of your soul with every failed diet program or every person who made you feel like it's your fault the diets don't work. I assure you, the system failed you; some might say your body failed you. But *you* did not fail. To succeed on this journey, you need to get to know yourself in order to avoid the pitfalls that hijack your success, and you need to adopt a vision and lifestyle that set you up for lifelong success. Do. Not. Skip. This. Chapter. It will set you up to achieve your goals. Let me be clear: working on mindset and your mental game does not mean that you are weak. It in fact means the opposite. I have come to appreciate that it takes a lot of mental strength to invest in my mindset and to keep myself primed for long-term success.

When you are truly getting to know yourself, there are some key concepts to consider:

- How susceptible are you to external influences?
- How do you form habits, and what kind of support systems do you need?
- Are you a rule follower or a rule breaker?
- How do you spend your time?
- How can you challenge yourself and push your limits to expand your success?

The work is going to be worth it. When you have the right program for your physiology and the right program for your mindset, you will be unstoppable!

Forming Habits and Keeping Accountable for Your Success

This section was inspired by one of my author girl crushes, Gretchen Rubin. She has a way of taking everything I know from working on myself and with patients and organizing it in a most approachable way. In Gretchen's book *Better than Before* (*Copyright 2015, Doubleday Canada*) she discusses key concepts that pertain to getting to know yourself. I love how she breaks these down not into right or wrong, but instead into being empowered by knowing your habit-forming style and your body. This is key to ongoing success.

The first concept Gretchen explores is establishing whether you are an abstainer or a moderator. Have you ever wondered how someone can have a chocolate bar stored at home and just eat one piece of it, whereas you would just choke that thing down in one sitting and need to have your house clear of temptations? Well, that's the difference between a moderator and an abstainer. For a long time, I thought that abstaining from a food, for example sugar, was the only way to go. I would set myself up for a challenge and deny myself any sugar. Then what would happen? You know it: all that I could think about was sugar. I would obsess over it, and use all of my willpower to white knuckle it to the end of the month. At the end of that month, I would eat all the things I had denied myself, and then beat myself up wondering why I even started in the first place.

If that scenario sounds familiar, you may also be a moderator. I think it's partially my years of restrictive dieting, but man, oh man, when you tell me I can't have something for a period of time or can't do something, that thing becomes the focus of my attention. In contrast, I can have a nice bar of dark chocolate at home in my cupboard and snack on it little by little over the course of a week. Knowing I can have just a small piece is enough to satiate my mind and my appetite for that thing.

Another component in Gretchen's book (*which really is a must-read*) is the concept of rules. Depending on your susceptibility and also your habit-forming styles, you will either be a lover of rules or a hater of rules. My system with rules takes something completely off the table, not for a month or a week but for good. This may sound drastic, but if you have a health issue or if you have a seriously addictive personality, this may be what you have to do. I cannot eat gluten because I have celiac disease. I have severe whole body symptoms if I eat gluten; therefore, it's just off the table for me. I don't think about gluten, dream about gluten, or miss gluten. It's just non-existent to me. I'm always asked, "Don't you wish you could have that bread? Wouldn't you eat it if you could?" And my answer is always no. Because it's just one of my rules, it occupies none of my willpower bucket or my mind. Some of you may need to make this rule with flour, grains, sugar, or dairy. You may need something set in stone that takes an option out of the ranks for good. It's possible that, for you, the idea of rules may be a huge relief instead of a burden. I have a lot of patients who feel this way. There's nothing quite like seeing someone fall into their stride with these strategies, because when you really get to know yourself, this is where the magic happens.

A warning about habit styles. If you are forcing yourself into one type or another, or wish you were a rule maker so you choose to adopt that style, it will do you more harm than good. For years, I thought it was sexy to be a rule maker and to be able to walk into a party or an event and simply state, "I don't eat sugar or grains" (in addition to all of my gluten-free requirements). Society has a way of glorifying those decisions or types of people, which is unfortunate. Every time I have said that and then eaten the sugar or grains, it takes a huge toll on my mindset and my belief about what's possible. There is nothing as damaging to your mindset as consistently breaking a promise with yourself or making choices that are not in line with your goals.

If you find you are heading home at the end of the night and beating yourself up about all of the missteps of the day, it's time to change your beliefs and rules and get to know yourself. When you push yourself into a box that doesn't fit you, you will likely rebel or hate yourself in the process, which in both cases beats down your willpower, your willingness to try again, and ultimately your success.

As a final note, it's critical to understand what accountability systems you need to have in place in order to get things done. Do you need community? A partner in crime to check in with? Do you just need information, and when you make a decision you drive forward on it? Do you rebel against instructions? Do you need a specific plan (i.e., a 30-day meal plan), or do you fare better with general guidelines (i.e., paleo eating)? I am well aware that I have likely just raised more questions than I have provided answers to, but no one can answer these except you. And when you do get the answers for yourself, it is powerful. Remember, none of these are right or wrong, one way is not better than another. It's all about what is right for you. I highly recommend you put some thought into your habits and accountability plan.

"IF YOU DO NOT KNOW HOW YOU'RE SPENDING YOUR TIME, YOU WILL NOT KNOW HOW TO BETTER INCORPORATE HEALTHY HABITS, SLEEP, STRESS REDUCTION, MEAL PREP, EXERCISE, OR ANYTHING ELSE INTO YOUR DAY."

How You Spend Your Time

If you do not know how you're spending your time, you will not know how to better incorporate healthy habits, sleep, stress reduction, meal prep, exercise, or anything else into your day. Knowing how my days are set up has helped to attach new habits to my current ones. For example, I want to add more exercise to my lifestyle, and I have a habit of waking up in the morning (don't we all?). I love exercising once I get to the gym, but I always think about the thousand things on my to-do list that I could get done during that hour. I know that if I'm going to work out that day I have to take a current habit I have, waking up, and attach it to what I want to do, going to the gym. Taking the action of the gym and tying it to waking up allows me to automate the whole process. I don't even think about it; I just roll out of bed and into the car.

Grace wanted to incorporate more HIIT into her day, but no matter where we tried to fit in that five minutes, she just kept skipping it. In this case I got creative. One of Grace's biggest loves in life is coffee; she just could not be without her morning java. I used this to my advantage. It takes about five minutes for a pot of coffee to fully brew, so we agreed that while her coffee brewed, instead of staring into the abyss awaiting that beautiful taste, Grace was going to do two push-ups, five squats, and five jumping jacks. This sounds like nothing, hardly qualifies for a work out, does it? But what I know is that the hardest part of establishing a habit is getting started. Once you get started, you can go all day. The key is making something seem so easy, so simple, that it feels ridiculous not to do it. And then you do it. Better yet, you keep going! Sure enough, she started with the simple exercises and within a week she was getting a full ten- to fifteen-minute HIIT training in more days than not, and on her days off, she made a deal with herself that she would still do the push-ups, squats, and jumping jacks just to keep the habit and to "earn" her coffee. Yes, that reward is critical as well.

Take Action
Using the workbook at **www.sarahwilsonnd.com/ loseitbookbonus**, take stock of what you are doing throughout the day and look for areas where you can attach new positive habits that feel too easy, so simple that anyone could accomplish them. The hardest part of establishing a new habit is finding a place to fit it into your day and the physical act of starting it. Once you do just one, say, push-up, you'll be surprised how easy it is to end up doing five, 10, or 15 more.

Food Cues

Understanding your day in terms of food is equally critical to breaking habit cycles. It's likely that in this exercise you will find there are reproducible cycles of cravings, desires, and appetite changes throughout the day. For example, while I was in medical school, for a long time the only break I had during the day was when I stopped for meals, which meant my meals were often in front of the TV. This created a cycle that indicated to my body that TV time meant food time. Even if I had just eaten, I would have cravings as soon as I sat down to watch a show. (This is a common habit for people to have to break, especially because I'm asking you not to eat after dinner, and that's the time of day most of us watch our favourite episodes.) Yes, sometimes those cravings would come from me not eating a healthy rounded dinner, but often it's that we get cues from our external environment. These cues are powerful: they tell us to eat at a specific time, to eat when we drive past a certain store, to have cravings when we see the food advertisements on TV. Recognizing these cues and either avoiding the triggers or resisting the urge to mistake them for hunger are essential to avoiding late-night, out of circadian timing eating. Not only is this strategy a critical piece to knowing yourself, but it's also a hack for avoiding pitfalls that hijack your success. More on that next.

Willpower Myth

Everything drains your willpower cup, it just depends on the rate at which it happens. Have you ever come home at the end of the day, been asked what you want for dinner, and had a complete meltdown? I mean "angry, indecisive, I shouldn't have to always make the decisions, this sucks, you suck, I suck, just make the decision, and fall face first into fast food because no one wants to make the decision" calibre meltdown? My poor husband can attest to this! Like you, all I do all day long is make decisions. Decisions about my business, how to treat patients, what to wear, what workout to do, the list goes on. One thing I try my best not to make decisions on anymore is food because decision fatigue drains our willpower and ability to make decisions that are in line with our goals.

There has been some interesting research done on willpower because, let's be honest, even the researchers want more of it! What they've discovered is that yes, consuming addictive, stimulating foods, such as gluten, dairy, and sweet fatty foods, drains our willpower. Other willpower zapping things include making decisions throughout the day, resisting temptation (i.e., resisting foods in the office, food advertisements), blood glucose fluctuations, and low blood glucose in general. This makes those evening cravings all the more difficult to resist. The best part of this research though is the discovery that we can actually refill the willpower bucket with specific activities. These things include gratitude journaling, prayer, meditation, social connection (with the right people), sleep, and glucose consumption.[99] No wonder so many of us have sugar cravings, especially at night!

Among all of these possibilities, connecting with my accountability partners, providing that social connection, and gratitude journaling are my non-negotiables. I will discuss gratitude journaling more later in this chapter, as it is one of my daily success habits. In the meantime, think about the most recent craving you've had, something that almost sent you into a nighttime eating spiral. What if, instead of eating, you took a bath and made a list of all the things you are truly grateful for? What you are grateful for about your current body, your health, your life, your safety, etc.? Would that craving have been as strong? Both my personal experience and the research suggest that cravings don't have as much of a hold on us in if we redirect our attention.

"IF YOU FAIL TO PLAN YOU PLAN TO FAIL."

Make a Plan

It probably comes as no surprise that most New Year's resolutions fail. They fail because people don't know why they want to achieve something, but perhaps even more because people neglect to plan. You can't just declare, "I am going to lose weight," and expect to will the change into existence. How are you going to make that happen? Will you exercise more, eat less? Okay, now what? When are you going to exercise? What are you going to do? How are you going to go, say, low carb? Will you buy a program or cookbook? What are you going to eat when you go out or when you're at a meeting? Having a plan not only sets you up to overcome the decision fatigue and the willpower gap, but it's also how you achieve goals. *If you fail to plan you plan to fail.*

When setting goals, a daily plan is far more important than the end result. For example, if my goal is to lose 10 lbs, I know I have to follow the diet laid out here. I know that I need to get more sleep and plan to start during a time when I don't have a lot of deadlines. I need to be able to plan regular meals, get to the gym, and really understand why those 10 lbs matter, because for me, my *why* is the thing that drives me above anything else.

I consult my planner, check to make sure that it's just my regular routine with no obstacles upcoming. Then I look at the meal plan, make shopping lists, and enlist my husband to help cook or at least forewarn him that things will be changing a bit. Then I write in my planner my gym time, travel time back and forth, meal prep times, bedtimes, and self-care times. These are non-negotiable, they are planned weeks to months in advance so that I don't have to make decisions about them in the moment (avoiding decision fatigue), and I don't let anyone book into these scheduled plans. Nothing except serious tiredness, a need for self-care, or an illness will get in my way. You can make time for anything else in the other hundred hours of the week. This is what needs to be scheduled: eight hours of sleep per night, plus one hour set aside for mealtimes, plus workouts and self-care.

"THE MOMENT THAT I REALIZED I WANTED TO BE HEALTHY BECAUSE I'M WORTH IT, BECAUSE I WANT TO GIVE MY EDUCATION, MY LIFE EXPERIENCE, AND MY PASSION TO THE WORLD, WAS THE MOMENT MY EXPERIENCE WITH HEALTH CHANGED."

Mindset, Visioning, and Lifestyle Design

Now that you're on your way to mastering the basics of habits and overcoming hijacks, we can get into the fun stuff. The mindset and lifestyle design piece is what lights me up. It's the list of things that I am continuously adding to and changing to up-level my health and my healthy lifestyle.

What do people do to achieve lifelong health, stick with their goals, and keep on track with the lifestyle that serves them the most? They live proactively. These successful patients, myself and some of the world's top achievers, do not live their life reacting to their environment. They set up their environment in such a way that they are ready for what life throws at them, taking it in stride in the context of their healthy lives.

Of course the goal with this book is to correct your insulin resistance, stabilize your hangry, and have you feeling emotionally stable between meals (even if there is an extra hour stuck in traffic before you can get that meal in). In any case, having a system where you plan in advance can ease the burden of making these changes. Start with planning what to eat. It doesn't matter whether that means meal prep a few times per week or you come home from the grocery store and clean all your vegetables so that when you get home at night it's all set for you. It's about choosing a path that works for you.

Planning when to eat is another critical component to structuring your environment for weight loss success. What I find is that most women in today's busy world don't have set mealtimes. How often do you eat on the run, between meetings, or worse, instead of meals you find yourself snacking throughout the day? Whether you are eating three meals per day, or fasting and eating two larger meals, you need to set mealtimes, commit to them, and eat within an hour of those times. This is critical for your circadian rhythm, as it primes your digestive system and metabolic system to be ready for food, and also it prepares your mind. When you know you'll be eating in a half hour, for example, you think about the type of food you'll be eating, you relax a bit, getting into your parasympathetic state, ready to take a break and eat. You look forward to it. All of these subtleties are important because they help to prepare our bodies and minds for success.

Scheduling mealtimes also prevents you from going eight hours without eating only to emerge from a work coma, starving, which can lead to late-night binging, eating whatever is close at hand, and as a result, bloating and gas, fatigue, blood sugar swings, and weight gain. I know, we've all done it. But let's make an effort to keep it at bay.

Self-Control versus Self-Care

The moment that I realized I wanted to be healthy because I'm worth it, because I want to give my education, my life experience, and my passion to the world, was the moment my experience with health changed. I know now that when I eat poorly or don't take care of my body, I end up with brain fog and zapped energy. This, to me, is selfish behaviour because when I'm not taking care of myself, I can't give my best to my patients, my family, or my writing, and that doesn't serve anyone. Now I approach healthy lifestyle changes from a place of self-care.

It's easy to buy into the system of what I call "sexy self-control", the belief that people who have the most discipline are the ones who are going to succeed; it's the widely held assumption that if you can starve yourself, if you have the willpower to work out for three hours a day, you are a better person. It's just ingrained in our society, isn't it? Feeling like your body is out of control, no matter what you eat or do, leads to a desperate drive to control something. You better believe that I'm on a mission to bust that myth wide open, because the sad reality is that one, two, five years later those women are in my office, suffering. They have taxed their adrenal glands, pushed their brain to exhaustion, damaged their metabolic hormones, and most often, affected their gut. They are coming to me, saying their "old tricks" to feel well or lose weight aren't working. There's just not enough coffee, they cannot go low carb enough, low calorie enough, or ramp up their workouts enough to prevent the weight from creeping back on. This is the epitome of the pursuit of health taking the form of self-control versus self-care. It's also why this book has so many sections, and why I'm not just saying treat your insulin resistance and move on, because after a while, individually these things don't work and you need to support your whole body.

For me, getting out of the mindset of "work harder, be more in control," really opened up my world. It allowed me to see what exercises worked well, what foods worked well, and in what space I felt my best. This is what I want for you as well. Once you recognize self-care as your key to success, you will get control of your life. It sounds counter-intuitive, but it's true. This mindset starts with personal development, reading this chapter, and other books, that challenge your thinking. It takes listening to your body and pushing your boundaries, trying things that make you uncomfortable, and stopping to breathe and take in life. It's about treating your life like an experiment, trying things, recording your responses, and broadening your horizons to what is possible.

I never thought that some days I would trade my spinning class for a long walk, or that I would fast and be able to go hours without food, effortlessly. For me, challenging my beliefs about what health should be was where the magic happened.

Take Action
If you are brutally honest with yourself, what is one thing you are doing out of self-control? Is it eating that cardboard-tasting bread? Running yourself into the ground with cardio? Throwing in the towel completely? None of those things truly come from a place of self-love and compassion. Challenge yourself to ditch one control item and add in one self-care item today!

"ALIGNMENT ISN'T ABOUT ACHIEVING A GOAL, IT'S ABOUT BEING ON THE PATH."

Make Decisions from Alignment and Identity Shift

As you start to change your lifestyle and your day-to-day habits, you will notice one of two things. You keep hitting obstacles with the changes or you change your view of yourself and find success much more streamlined. The difference between these paths is your view of yourself and your identity. It's very common when you have struggled with weight loss resistance for a long time to take on the identity of a failure, someone who is destined to be overweight. Not all but some of my patients have gone so far as to say that for years they felt like people looked at them as if they were lazy and ate poorly; therefore, they just accepted the identity of someone who does not care for themselves. This is a dangerous place to make commitments and agreements out of because it's completely disempowered. This is where a slow but sure "fake it until you make it" identity change is required for any kind of long-term success.

What is the identity that you currently hold on to?

Now, what is the identity that you wish you held?

When you make decisions from the identity of someone who's empowered and self-loving, when you at least *act* as if you were that person, it can be easier to make decisions about what to do, eat, and how to act from a place of alignment. Alignment means you are consistent, not deviating from the path toward your goals. Everything you're doing comes from the same space and perspective. Alignment comes with honouring yourself and gives you that feeling of achievement you get after, say, you've done a great workout and eaten a super healthy breakfast. It's a stark contrast between that person and the person who emotionally eats too much chocolate cake. We all know those feelings of remorse, regret, and frustration; the feelings of making choices that are out of alignment with our goals and identity. Alignment isn't about achieving a goal, it's about being on the path.

Some of you reading this are undoubtedly thinking, *Okay lady, I came here for action and diet changes, not this mindset crap.* And to all of you, I used to be there, and I hear you. This seems like the last thing that would work to help you achieve your goals. There's no question that you can take the action strategies in the beginning of the book and see massive results. But please remember this section when you're struggling and still feel as if you have that last 10–15% to go or when you feel like you're having to force yourself through the process. When you are ready, this mindset chapter will be here.

Take Action

To help solidify your vision and your alignment, take some time to journal (write or record yourself talking) about the identity you want to hold. Then come up with some affirmations, things you can read to yourself, things you can program into the calendar on your phone to pop up, to remind you of the identity you want to align with.

Develop a New Baseline

If you truly want to ditch the "on the wagon, off the wagon" mindset, develop a new baseline. It's taken me years of trial and error, but when patients get it and embrace it, their lives change overnight.

Picture this: you come back from vacation, you've got "airplane flu," your work email has exploded in your absence, and the world suddenly seems chaotic. You feel overwhelmed and the last thing you can think about is diet and lifestyle. What are the foods you fall back on and what is the lifestyle you choose? This is your baseline. For me, that has changed drastically; my baseline now is vegetables. When all else fails, I will throw together a bowl of veggies (fresh, frozen, whatever is in my kitchen, but my kitchen is always stocked). I know that I can smother them in fat and spices and I have a five-minute meal that keeps me feeling full and my brain and waistline on point. That is what I mean by a new baseline. My baseline lifestyle is no longer takeout from a processed food restaurant. It may be a salad from a quality place, or fresh veggies from a local restaurant, but quality remains at the forefront. The same is true of exercise. If I'm feeling far too exhausted to go do a HIIT workout or head to the gym, then I still head out for a long walk, listening to a podcast or my favourite soundtrack.

Pre-planning strategies for life's eventualities is critical to success:

- How are you going to take care of yourself if you lose sleep?
- How are you going to ensure you can rest and not fall into the craving cycle?
- What are you going to eat when chaos ensues?
- Do you have local restaurants, frozen meals, or meal delivery services that offer quality options?
- What are your baseline movement activities?

"RESEARCH HAS SHOWN THAT GRATITUDE HELPS US LIVE LONGER, MAKE BETTER CHOICES, HAVE STRONGER RELATIONSHIPS, AND WARD OFF THE EFFECTS OF STRESS ON THE BODY."

Gratitude Journaling

What do you have to be grateful for? It seems a simple question, but what if I asked you to make a list, every single day, of the things you were grateful for? It can be a challenge, especially because we are primed to look for danger, to respond to the negative things happening in our days. This is our ancestral genes and neurological system trying to alert us to all the stuff that can take us down. We don't really respond so much to the amazing moments that we can use to reframe our days. Between the negative news portrayed and the fear-based advertising, who has the mental space to commit to looking for moments to be grateful for? No one does, if they don't make time.

It's easy to get caught up in the minutia of life. We wake up, start our day in likely the most reactive way possible, get to work, respond to all the tasks at hand, take a break for lunch if we're lucky, finish the day, workout if we're lucky, eat dinner, spend time in the evening with friends and family, rush everyone to sleep, trying to wind down before crashing, wiped from the day. Then we get up and start it all again. That doesn't sound very inspiring. That is, until you look for the moments to be grateful for. Gratitude journaling has taken me from that place on the hamster wheel into waking up grateful for the day, for all the people I get to help, for my health, for my husband, and my family. I walk through the day looking for the things to celebrate in my life, come home grateful for all that I have accomplished, and for the opportunity to learn, grow, move my body, and fuel it in the best way I can. Research has shown that gratitude helps us live longer, make better choices, have stronger relationships, and ward off the effects of stress on the body.[100,101] All things that you need if you are reading this book.

One app that I love for this is the Five Minute Journal by Intelligent Change. You can also use my specific gratitude journal in the workbook, found at **www.sarahwilsonnd.com/loseitbookbonus**. I bet you'll find yourself not only having a different perspective on your day, but gratitude journaling also primes you to look for moments to be grateful for.

Pave Your Path with Priming

People who succeed with lifestyle changes decide to. They decide that their past health struggles are not their future health struggles. They decide that they will dictate the course of their lives, and they will not let small setbacks overwhelm, or their negative mental chatter and fears get in the way. When I was trying to "mind over matter" my way through my fear of failure to make yet another lifestyle change, I used affirmations and priming to fake it at first. What does this look like? Well, I had affirmative sayings like, you will be successful or you are beautiful, deserving and strong, all over my bathroom mirror, as pop-ups on my phone, and as a journal entry that I made and repeated to myself every day. Did I believe it? No way! And I certainly felt awkward and fraudulent early on as I read these things. But I committed to my word until I started to believe it. Even now, when I am facing fear, overwhelm, and am tackling a new goal, I will go back to these habits and start setting myself up for what I want to achieve.

Similarly, I *strongly* believe in the power of *priming*, a positive psychology term that describes the act of paving the path before you walk along it. Priming, in the way that I teach it, can take different forms. You can pave your entire journey where you set out all the milestones and step-by-step things you're going to take to keep you motivated along the way. This also helps you to see how your daily actions are directly related to the goal you have for months down the road.

Another way to set up priming is at the end of each day, plan out your next day. What would make tomorrow a successful day? You can also do this the morning of, but realistically a lot of us rush through the mornings and forget to attend to this. Are you going to go to the gym, move your body, grocery shop, meal prep? Are you going to take a self-care time out? Are you going to finally finish changing up your home environment to reflect the lifestyle you want? You check in, in the morning, to set the stage for what you want your day to look like, and then reflect back at night to see if those tasks were completed; it reinforces your health journey. This approach also helps take decision fatigue out of your daily equation.

The Finally Lose It Mindset Review

- Your success is not going to occur by accident. It's calculated, planned, and proven to help you reach your goals. Rebooting your mindset is an essential component to recovering your metabolic health. Overlooking your mindset is why most diet books fail to help anyone in the long term.
- You truly need to become a student of self-improvement when you step into habit change and a lifestyle level up. I can't promise that the journey will feel effortless in the beginning, but I've witnessed that it does pay off in the end!
- You will discover, just as I did, that finding yourself through personal development, redefining your day, your habits, and your thought patterns will bring you as much success and contentedness as losing excess weight.

PART TWO

The Finally Lose It Action Plan

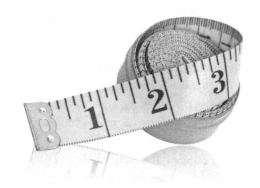

A s we begin to dive into the action plan it's a fine time to review the rules of the program (which first appear on **page 20**). Please reread these before moving on to the diet and lifestyle implementation plans.

The Rules of Engagement

The Finally Lose It Program

Say yes to:

Stocking whole foods. Delicious, simple, easy to find whole foods.

Thinking about when and how you eat. As much as diet, i.e., the foods you choose, is a cornerstone of this plan, when and how you eat are also critical factors in overcoming your weight loss resistance. This book teaches you how to personalize timing and approach to meals in the Finally Lose It Program.

Personalizing your plan. Everything in this program needs to be customized to you. That is why you find quizzes throughout the book and a laboratory blood work guide at the back so that you can work with a medical practitioner to get to the bottom of your health concerns.

Getting adequate sleep and reducing stress. Frankly, you need to be taught how important quality sleep and stress reduction are if you want to meet your goals and sustain your progress. Many women are never taught how to reduce their stress or support their sleep; these are foundational pieces to the Finally Lose It Program.

Checking your mindset. Adopt a growth mindset. Accept new challenges. Look at how you have gone about weight loss in the past, and change your views and your habits. These elements are not often discussed in weight loss books, but they have proven to be pivotal to the ongoing success of every woman who has been through the Finally Lose It Program.

Say no to:

A "no pain, no gain" mentality. This program is not hard. I promise you have been through much harder things in life, even much harder programs. When you are stressed to the nines and then you add the stress of another fad diet, it's no wonder that you don't see the results you have hoped for. Weight loss doesn't have to be painful.

Making excuses. Excuses, simply put, are broken promises to yourself. They offer nothing except a feeling of failure and incompetence. Over time, you have likely learned to take them on as opportunities for your mindset gremlins to step in and prove to you that you can't do it, you aren't good enough, and that you shouldn't try again. Lose these excuses on Day 1. In Finally Lose It you will work with your habit forming type. You will not feel suffocated by this health plan and we offer accountability to boot.

Eating cardboard "diet" food. You never have to eat tasteless, funky ingredient-filled, gross food anymore. I mean it! Don't eat food that you do not like. Don't like Brussels sprouts? Don't eat them! When food becomes a forced experience, you will never sustain the results, and you will crave more junk foods.

Eating inflammatory and addictive foods. Sugar, artificial sweeteners, industrial seed oils, food additives, alcohol, wheat, dairy, and grains will be cut out for 30 days in phase 3. These foods interact with your brain to aggravate cravings, and they also can cause inflammation in your brain, gut, and metabolic system. Both of these factors, cravings and inflammation, exacerbate weight loss resistance.

Complicated shopping lists, meal plans, and overwhelming meal prep. There are few things that frustrate me more than a shopping list four pages long, spending hours in the grocery store looking for obscure ingredients, and spending hundreds of dollars at the cash register, only to get home to use 1 tsp. of an ingredient, and then the rest ends up going bad. I have developed a system for meal preparation that focuses on delicious ingredients, simple preparation, and a shopping list that fits on a Post-it note!

LET THY **FOOD** BE THY **MEDICINE** AND **MEDICINE** BE THY **FOOD.**

—HIPPOCRATES

8

LET'S TALK ABOUT FOOD

This book would not be a wellness, health, or weight loss book without a chapter on food and meal planning. This is because what you eat sets the foundation for your health, and your results. Food really can be medicine. The issue I have is that today food is more often used as a punishment or reward system, especially when it comes to weight loss. How many times have you resigned yourself to dry chicken breast and broccoli, cabbage soup, or worse, processed and packaged foods that have no nutritional value? These are fads, they are short term, nutrient deficient, and they set you up for cravings, failure, and teach you very little about your body. Here, though, things are different.

My goal is for every woman to leave this book knowing what a healthy diet looks like for herself. I want you to know how many servings of protein, carbohydrates, fat, and fibre you can eat to lose weight and feel great. I also want you to learn how to look at food simply, to meal prep and take the stress out of nourishing food. It is about personalizing your plan, which should come as no shock at this point. That's how you will reach your goals and be able to sustain the results.

How to Use this Chapter

Now that we are in the action section, I want to give you a map of how to best navigate the plan. When I am walking patients through this method, we always spend time discussing the foundational food qualities that you need to overcome weight loss resistance. It is no surprise for me to hear "Dr. Sarah, can you just tell me what to do please?" when we are halfway through. I promise that will happen, but first I have to set the stage! Right after you learn why you are choosing the foods you are and get a primer on how I implement successful meal prep, you will take a quiz to help you identify the best phase for you to start on. After that, read the associated phase, decide if you want to DIY (do it yourself) or follow the set out system. Then make a plan and dive in. You will be in this phase one to two weeks before moving to the next phase. If you feel hangry, have a lot of cravings, get cold, tired or are just struggling to get started then stay in your initial phase for one extra week before moving on to the next phase.

Foundational Food Principles

The Finally Lose It system follows principles of nutrient density, polyphenol and fibre richness, satiety, low insulin demand, and macronutrient balance. It's psychologically compatible (treats or no treats), flexible, offering fasting days and carb complement days, and perhaps best of all, it's simple to execute.

Nutrient Density

Nutrient density is important when you are trying to lose weight because you need to fit a whole lot of nutrients into less food volume. Nutrient density also ensures that your cravings are not coming from being low on a specific nutrient. With this diet, you can say goodbye to your multivitamin; you're going to get all that you need and more from your food.

Polyphenol Content

As you've seen from **chapter 5**, polyphenols are important for reducing metabolic endotoxemia, improving insulin sensitivity, and balancing blood sugar. We are also coming to understand that polyphenols are important for the function of mitochondria, your energy-producing powerhouses. At 2,000 mg (2 g) per day, you will improve your energy, your insulin signalling, and optimize your gut health.

Satiety

Satiety is the feeling of fullness you experience after you eat a meal. Staying full is obviously critical to reducing cravings, eating a reasonable amount at meals, and extending your fast between meals. I find that incorporating satiating foods into your diet is especially important when you have yo-yo dieted, have altered gut hormone signalling, and insulin resistance. These states predispose us to feeling hungry 24-7.

Research studies help us understand which foods will keep us feeling full the longest. The most notable study was done by Susanna Holt.[102] She used white bread, a widely accepted satiating food, and compared other foods to that in terms of how much participants chose to eat and drink and how they felt for two hours after. Although this is a small study, a lot can be gleaned from it. White potatoes, for example, are the most satiating food. These have long been deemed the devil's spawn in the weight loss community, but no longer. Yes, white potatoes have a significant insulin response, which we need to monitor, but there's no reason to eliminate them from the diet. Other relevant satiating foods included in this study were ling/cod fish, oranges, apples, grapes, beef, beans, eggs, lentils, and rice. Although only 38 foods were studied, an equation was made to help apply the findings of this and other studies on satiety to other commonly consumed foods. This equation is what I have used to help fill you up with the most satiating vegetables, fruits, meat, fat, and starches. No more hangry days!

Hunger versus Cravings
Many women don't actually know the feeling of true hunger because the most common hunger signals are cravings. If you are weight loss resistant, your hormonal signalling is all kinds of messed up and your body and brain are doing their best to try to differentiate what everything means. Try drinking a large glass of lemon water with some chia seeds if you think you are having cravings and not true hunger. This is the perfect combination of hydration, fibre and a sour flavour that can curb empty cravings.

Fibre Content

Fibre is critical for health from so many different angles. Your beneficial flora, or bacteria, depend on proper fibre consumption in order to grow and produce the short-chain fatty acids that your gut lining needs. Fibre also helps to eliminate excess cholesterol, hormones, and toxins in your poop. Not to mention all the benefits to gut hormone signalling, insulin and glucose, and satiety that we've already explored.

North Americans consume a lot less fibre than they need. The USDA claims the average fibre intake is 16 g per day. This is in stark contrast to the 45 g that I like to see people get daily! No wonder constipation and digestive issues are prevalent.

Word of warning: increase your fibre slowly. If you jump from 15 g to 45 g overnight, you will shock your system and experience bloating, gas, and distension. The upcoming meal plans will guide you to slowly increase your fibre intake; phase 3 is set up for at least 45 g of fibre. If you opt to jump into this phase, I recommend that you increase your added fibre (chia, flax, hemp hearts, inulin, psyllium) by 1–3 tsp. at a time.

Low Insulin Demand

The food insulin demand (FID) has been a helpful construct for me to design a diet that goes far beyond the low-carb, low insulin understanding. If I went back to my macro eating, bodybuilding-style meal plans, I would surely gain weight again. We have come to understand that it's not only carbohydrates that stimulate insulin, but too much protein, dairy, and fatty sweet foods are also culprits. In phase 1 and phase 2, we'll be starting to limit your consumption of dairy, grains, and all refined carbohydrates. You will have enough protein to keep you feeling full, enough to maintain and develop your lean muscle mass, but not enough to drive your insulin over the top. (For most women, this puts them in the range of 90–120 g of protein per day.) You will also notice that snacking will be eliminated. Cutting dairy out of your diet—yes, dairy—will not only lower your insulin response, but it can also lower your inflammation levels. Most adults do not tolerate dairy well. Once we can break through your casomorphin addiction, you will likely agree.

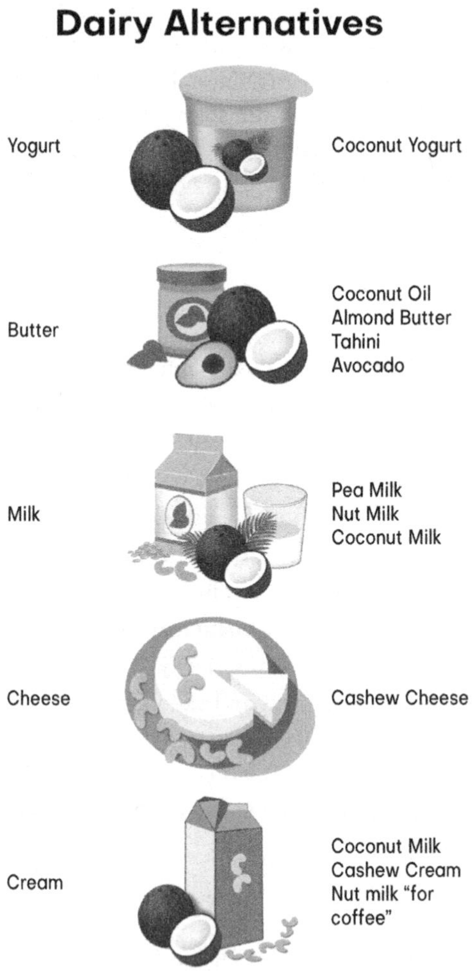

Dairy Alternatives

Yogurt		Coconut Yogurt
Butter		Coconut Oil Almond Butter Tahini Avocado
Milk		Pea Milk Nut Milk Coconut Milk
Cheese		Cashew Cheese
Cream		Coconut Milk Cashew Cream Nut milk "for coffee"

Figure 18. This image provides Finally Lose It–approved alternatives to dairy. These easy swaps will make your switch to a dairy-free lifestyle seamless.

What about the Calcium?

Repeat after me: dairy alone does not protect your bones. If this were the case, surveys would not have shown that the highest dairy consuming countries also have some of the highest rates of osteoporosis. (I bet that shocked you!) Dairy is a convenient source of calcium for many people, but your bone density is determined by genetics, exercise, smoking, alcohol, weight, hormones, and vitamin D status as well. So yes, calcium is a critical nutrient, but it can be obtained through a whole foods, no-dairy diet.

The average woman needs between 600 and 1,000 mg of calcium throughout the day. This is not a massive amount when looking at a whole foods meal plan such as the one I have created. For instance, one serving of shrimp has 15% of your daily requirements; two servings of leafy greens as much as 10%. Most milk alternatives are also fortified to include added calcium, making up as much as 50% of your required intake. Needless to say, your calcium needs will be covered.

A Case for Fasting

Understanding insulin is not just about how much your body makes immediately after a meal, but also what happens between meals and overnight. As discussed, if you are snacking throughout the day, you are constantly in a fat-storing mode. The same is true if insulin runs high overnight. And if your insulin is perpetually high at the moment, you will need to go low and slow with fasting. Fasting allows more time for insulin levels to get into the ideal range (See appendix A for lab values.) and supports proper insulin signalling. If you can tolerate even a 12–14-hour fast, it will speed up your progress, as your high insulin can contribute to more difficulty in accessing your fat for fuel. (Remember, insulin locks your fat cells and makes your body want to use sugar as fuel.) Being dependent on sugar results in feeling hangry and overwhelmed between meals, and it spikes your stress hormone, cortisol. As discussed in **chapter 4**, blood sugar swings are a huge source of stress on the body.

Therefore, if you are currently grazing or snacking your way through the day, you will start in phase 1 by switching your snacks to low insulin–stimulating foods. These include a handful of nuts, berries, a *fat bomb,* or something like guacamole with celery, broccoli, peppers, or cucumbers. As you move into phase 3, you will see discussion of overnight fasting. No matter what phase you are on, I would like to see you achieving a 12-hour fast from dinner to breakfast. For some, this is enough time to reset the metabolic hormones and kick the body into fat-burning mode. A lower carb, moderate protein (low insulin demand) breakfast can also help to extend this, allowing you to get into fat-burning mode between meals.

If you are anything like me though, after 12 hours you will still experience sub-optimal fasting insulin levels. In the past, mine were double what they should be! What I have had to do for myself, and with patients, is begin to extend that 12-hour fasting window, ever so slowly, to a 14- or 16-hour window a few days per week. This may sound totally unapproachable, especially if you are eating every two to three hours. This is where that growth mindset comes in. Never would I have thought that I could fast 16 (or more) hours. I took baby steps into the fasting waters, and I not only survived but also I'm better for it on the other side.

Remember, if you are feeling burnt out or get exhausted, fasting longer than 12 hours might not be for you right now. Start with addressing your stress first.

Note of caution: for the purposes of this book, I do not recommend that you go beyond 16 hours of fasting. If you are burnt out or have significant metabolic hormone imbalances, you could live the whole day in fight or flight mode and become hypoglycemic. This is not ideal for anyone's physiology. If you feel the need to extend your fast for any reason, you should be under the care of a healthcare practitioner and get some testing done first.

Psychologically Compatible

I truly believe that our diets need to be compatible with our physiology and with our psychology. Most people don't meet their health goals because of the process it takes to get there. They find diets too restrictive, illogical, too complicated, or too hindering to their social lives. For the most part, this is a completely accurate finding. A healthy diet can look so different from person to person.

An example of setting up a plan that's psychologically compatible is whether or not you have "off plan" days. Note that I do not call them "cheat days"; there is no morality here, ladies! Some of you may feel that you are boxed into this meal plan or diet outline, and it will make you feel crazy. Even as you read this chapter, you may be thinking, I just can't give up my Saturday night date meal with my partner. You may be hesitant to start, or you may even resist making diet changes because you want to have some semblance of normalcy in your life and not feel too restricted. In this case, having a planned day when you get to go out and "live your life" may be the way to go. *Planned* is key, though. When you plan a day off, you can ensure that you are enjoying it and using it to mentally fulfill you.

Off days are also important if you're finding that a lower carbohydrate diet is causing you to feel sluggish and cold (see appendix B for how to monitor this). However, if your off plan meals turn into off plan days, and you end up hating yourself for your choices, you will likely fare better to stick to the plan as I've set it up for at least 30 days. If you are highly insulin resistant, or if you are highly responsive to the dopamine hit that comes with higher carb, higher fat meals, then cravings for those foods after an off plan meal will also work against you. In these cases, you're better served to endure the cravings (and redirect your attention to something like a hot bath or a long walk instead) so that you can experience food freedom in the end.

Finally, knowing your psychological susceptibility to "healthy treats" is critical to finding your balance with any lifestyle plan. If you tend to have an addictive personality, meaning you have a history of food addiction, drug addiction, alcohol abuse, or exercise abuse, for instance, then hold this as your warning. I have seen patients with this tendency often stumble into the trap of healthy treat abuse. What do I mean by a healthy treat? This is all the recipes online for paleo/keto/ Atkins/low-carb cookies, cakes, chocolate, bread, buns and muffins. If you are going out of your way to find these things or have already been planning how to replace that morning coffee and a muffin with a low-carb weight loss resistance– appropriate muffin, you absolutely should not engage in any treat making, because you are not breaking the pattern of addiction; you are just swapping these foods for a lesser evil. In this scenario it's not even about the food. It's about the psychology, the mindset, and the thought process. Just as we would never advise an alcoholic to swap beer for vodka, I would like to see you abstain from even the healthy treats for a full 30 days so that you can see the change in your mindset and your thought patterns around food.

If you have restricted foods for years and felt deprived, then it's going to be natural for you to want to overindulge. When this continues, when you still have cravings and a tendency toward overeating or binging on these foods after allowing them back into your life for weeks, we know that taking a psychological assessment of your food plan is necessary. Maybe you do draw the line that you're just the person who doesn't eat treats, sugar, etc. If that works for you, own it! It's all about knowing yourself and using these strategies to discover what the best long-term plan is for you.

Macronutrient Balanced

A long-term approach to health and weight loss does not include a no-carb, no-fat, or high-protein diet. They work for a while, for someone out there, but these are what I like to call therapeutic diets, not lifestyles. Just as you only take a medication for a specific purpose, for a set period of time, these diets should not be used consistently without good data driven reasons. So what am I recommending? You'll come to find out I won't ever recommend eliminating all fruit, for example, but instead swapping bananas, which are pure sugar, for berries that contain a ton of polyphenols and fibre. I recommend swapping pasta for high-fibre, low-carb options (such as bean pastas) that are used strategically in your week. It is about establishing a healthy baseline of lower carb, moderate fat, and moderate protein intake meals that are in sync with your body's rhythms and timed to your specific physiology. It is also about eating enough. I believe the minimum caloric intake should be 1,600 kcal for a lightly active person. Many of you will need more than this as your hormones come on line, but don't worry about counting calories here. All of this will be factored into the meal plans in **chapter 9** and into the DYI Meal Map serving sizes.

Simple to Execute: Do You Assemble or Do You Design?

Are you a food assembler or a gourmet recipe maker? Many of us aspire to cook elaborate, healthy, social media worthy meals, setting the bar unrealistically high. The reality is that enticing cookbooks and complex recipes are great, but they take time. That's why I find understanding the difference between recipe cooking and food assembling to be key.

I work with busy professional women and I understand that time constraints are one of the biggest factors that keep them from achieving their goals. That is why I advocate for assembling with no fussing, measuring, or dirtying heaps of dishes. It's simple, you take a protein, some veggies, some fat, some fibre, and throw it together with a spice or two and out the door you go. This difference may seem subtle to you, but let's test that. How would you feel if I asked you to make a beef stroganoff on a Wednesday night after a long day at work? Maybe overwhelmed? Now what about this:

Vegetables	Protein	Fat	Fibre	Spice/Polyphenol
Mushrooms Onion Zucchini noodles	Beef strips	Coconut milk Coconut oil to fry	Coconut flour Garlic	Salt Pepper

Instructions: Put beef in a pan on low with coconut oil, onion, salt, and pepper. Cook 10 minutes. Add coconut flour and stir. Add the rest of the ingredients. Cook on low for 20 minutes.

The thought of a gourmet salad is overwhelming, but you can literally throw ingredients into a bowl and have a delicious, healthy meal in minutes.

Vegetables	Protein	Fat	Ferment	Spice/Polyphenol	Fruit
Spinach Pepper Tomato	Boiled eggs	Olive oil (and apple cider vinegar)	Kimchi	Herb salt Side of blueberries	Avocado

When you have the right pantry staples, and spend just an extra hour on a Sunday prepping, your week's meal preparations can be made seamless. I find just changing your mindset about food prep can make it easier when you are simply throwing ingredients into a pan.

Freedom and Lifestyle Focused

When you get the hang of this food system, you too will feel the benefits of the free-dom-focused, lifestyle-designed, and sustainable approach. No time to eat? You can fast for 16 hours until you have time to prepare something healthy. Having dinner at your Italian, or in my case Latino, in-laws? Then eat the carbs at that meal, just watch your serving sizes and call it your off day.

If you need more guidance, you can also strictly follow the meal plan and not have to think about anything, except the great feeling you are experiencing. You can feel mentally stable, lose weight, keep it off, and feel like yourself again—maybe even better than the best self you can remember, if you're anything like many of my patients. This plan truly has transformed my life and the life of countless others. I am excited for it to do the same for you.

Finally Lose It Meal System

Shopping and Meal Prep

Just like I believe in simple meal prep, I also believe in simple meal planning, for multiple reasons. The first reason is that research shows when the novelty is elim-inated from food and food is kept simple, study participants were better able to realize when they were full and eat only to that point. Having simple meals with common ingredients also helps to eliminate intense cravings, and when following this system, I see many patients able to sustain their weight loss longer. This is not only due to the effects on satiety, but I believe it's also because fewer ingredient and prep choices will decrease your decision fatigue.

Previously, I spoke about the fact that one of my success strategies was devel-oping a new baseline, where, if I'm busy and run home late, I will serve up a plate of vegetables, cover it in fat, and keep my blood sugar stable while I decide if I'm hungry enough to cook a protein or make something more substantial. The way that I do this is to ensure I always have similar ingredients in the house. That way I never have to make too many decisions or think about what to eat to the point that I end up with accidental takeout. The system we will explore below will help you to implement these same strategies.

As you saw in the Rules of Engagement, I have a disdain for extremely large shopping lists and three-hour marathons at the grocery store. I have heard many a patient echo that same sentiment. Combine that aversion with the research on nov-elty and decision fatigue and *ta-da*, we have the simple Finally Lose It meal system.

If you are following the meal plans provided then never fear, you are all set up. But if you want to go DIY, then this is how to create your own plan:

In each of the three phases of the meal plan, you will be given a DYI Meal Map. This lists the categories of foods and how many servings to eat per day within that category. This list is also available in printable format at **www.sarahwilsonnd.com/ loseitbookbonus**. You fill out the Finally Lose It meal map blank template, filling in each category (see below). You will select five vegetables, four different fibre and polyphenols, three different proteins and spices, two fermented foods, two fats, and one fruit on hand for the week. That's your weekly shopping list. If you are eating a dairy or a starch that will be added to the list, along with some pantry items the first time you shop. For one full week you will use just those ingredients to make completely different meals.

5-4-3-2-1 Weekly Shopping List

Vegetable					
Polyphenol					
Fibre					
Protein					
Spice					
Fat					
Fermented Food					
Fruit					
Starch					
Grain					
Dairy					

Pantry Staples and Stocking Up

In addition to the recipes and ingredients to be purchased for each phase, there's a list of pantry items that are helpful to have on hand. These will be used in the meal plan of each phase and can be added to recipes to change them up or season to your liking. They can also be found as a printout at **www.sarahwilsonnd.com/ loseitbookbonus**.

Pantry Staples for All Phases

Oils and Condiments
Olive oil
Avocado oil
Coconut oil
Apple cider vinegar
Balsamic vinegar
Lemon juice
Coconut aminos
Dijon mustard
Salt
Pepper
Coconut milk, full-fat (can)
Vanilla extract
Cocoa powder

Fibres
Hemp hearts
Ground flax seed
Chia seeds

Grains and Starches
Quinoa
Dried legumes of choice (black-eyed peas, kidney beans, chickpeas, pinto beans, etc.)

Pantry Nuts
Nuts (cashews, almonds, pumpkin seeds, sunflower seeds)

High polyphenol nuts (Chestnuts, hazelnuts, pecans)
Almond butter
Coconut flour

Beverages
Vegan Protein Powder
Stevia
Tea (herbal, green, and black)
Coffee
Coconut milk (carton)
Almond milk

About Beverages

During this program, I encourage you to drink at least eight to 10 cups of water, sparkling water, or herbal tea each day. Caffeinated tea and coffee, although allowed and encouraged, do not count as hydration. Drinking enough water is important for your digestion, skin health, energy, and to ward off cravings. Do not leave this out!

How much coffee is too much is a question I am asked frequently. So long as you are not feeling exhausted after drinking coffee, one to two cups of black coffee per day can be health promoting. Coconut or almond milk can be added, although sugar and cream should not.

Remember, coffee should not be consumed after 2:00 p.m. as it can affect your sleep and circadian rhythm.

Reintroduction of Foods

After the four weeks of the plan, the first thing people often ask about is the reintroduction of other fruits, grains, and starchy vegetables (because dairy is out for a while longer). My advice is to play to your tolerance. If you are losing weight, have increased energy, and decreased brain fog, inflammation, and gut symptoms, and then you add back in banana or dates, for example, and feel worse or your weight loss slows, then you should wait at least another two weeks before trying to increase those carbohydrates again. It can take up to three months to start to reset insulin resistance and make lasting changes to hormones and your circadian rhythm, and to affect change in other hormones. If you experience any sort of setback from reintroducing these foods, try reintroductions to your tolerance later on or stick to variations of the plan until you achieve your goals.

In appendix B there's also a guide to monitoring your blood glucose. If you are like the majority of those who have gone through this plan, you're going to want hard facts! In this case, as you are doing food reintroductions you can test your blood glucose before and after the meal. If your glucose is spiking higher than 7 mmol/L (126 mg/dL) at any point, or remains higher than 6 mmol/L (108 mg/dL) two hours after the meal, then that food is not working for you.

Note: as much as blood glucose doesn't make you gain weight, we don't have an at-home insulin meter at this point, so this is the best option we have.

What You Prepare For, You Can Achieve

Before we dive into your meal plan, here are some quick tips that help with meal preparation. First and foremost, batch cook and prepare in advance. When you go shopping, on a Sunday for example, make sure to set aside time for washing produce and prepping meals as well. In our house, we try to prepare food, especially our proteins, twice per week and then store them for easy access. Sunday and Thursday are those days. We will make our seasoned meats, our stews, or pot meals and then portion them out for the week. This is also a good time to wash and pre-chop vegetables. You can even pre-chop onions, peppers, mushrooms, cabbage, broccoli and cauliflower and have them ready for a whole month!

Take Action
I have a local market that sells produce pre-cut and frozen. The extra few dollars is so worth it to me! You may be asking, what about frozen? Yes, flash-frozen fruit, veggies, and even meats are A-OK, so long as you know the quality of those items was good before they were frozen.

Identify Your Finally Lose It Program Meal Phase

You are all coming into this book with different diets and drastically different understandings of what constitutes the best diet. Some of you have also likely given up on the whole issue until now, and are currently eating whatever you want because you've come to believe it apparently doesn't matter to your health goals anyway. Now is the time to customize the Finally Lose It approach even further. The following quiz will help you to establish whether you should start at phase 1 or phase 2, or if you are ready to dive right into phase 3.

Quiz: Determine Your Beginning Phase

How often do you eat throughout the day?
    a. Every two to three hours (three meals and two to three snacks) or tend to graze instead of eat meals.
    b. Three meals and one snack.
    c. Three meals only.

How do you feel if you are forced to skip a meal?
    a. Shaky, overwhelmed, weak, or hangry. I don't let that happen.
    b. Hungry! I would avoid it if I could and will try to find a snack.
    c. Fine, it happens. I get annoyed, but not from the hunger.

How often do you eat dairy (milk, cream, cheese, yogurt, etc.)?
    a. Daily.
    b. A few times per week, at least every other day.
    c. Never. I have cut out dairy.

How often do you eat grains (bread, pasta, flour ingredients)?
    a. Daily. I don't avoid any carbs.
    b. I don't eat a lot of grains, but I eat a lot of carbohydrates such as starchy carbs, legumes, and fruit.
    c. I eat low carb, so I generally avoid them.

What is your relationship with fat?
    a. I eat low fat and look for low-fat or reduced-fat items.
    b. I don't necessarily avoid fat, but I know it's high in calories, so I eat less of it.
    c. All of the good fats please! No fat fear here.

How many hours are there between your last bite of food at night and your first in the morning?
    a. I have a snack before bed and eat breakfast as soon as I wake up.
    b. I eat a late dinner, and then eat when I wake up, 8–10 hours.
    c. I avoid snacking after dinner, at least 12 hours.

How do you tolerate fibre?

    a.   I don't add fibre or know how much I eat.

    b.   I don't tolerate it well, I tend to avoid it.

    c.   I am totally fine with fibre, and eat a lot of it.

Do you have a lot of bloating, gas, abdominal pain, and inflammation?

    a.   I can at times.

    b.   Yes! Gut issues are definitely involved with my weight loss resistance.

    c.   Nope, I am totally fine in that area.

How Did You Score?

Mostly a's. You should start at phase 1. Here you will still be eating snacks throughout the day with some grains and dairy. A 12-hour fast is the goal here, so no snacking after dinner. I am going to get you comfortable with eating more fat and help to stabilize your blood sugar before moving into phase 2 after one week.

Mostly b's. You should start at phase 2. Say goodbye to your dairy, and grains are more limited here as well. In phase 2 you will not be snacking and we will focus on getting at least a twelve- to fourteen-hour overnight fast. In phase 2 there is an emphasis on slightly more fibre and fat, but not enough that it should aggravate metabolic endotoxemia and gut inflammation. If you're feeling well after one week in phase 2, move to phase 3. If not, stay here longer.

Do not move on to phase 3 before starting to treat gut issues. *If you are breast-feeding, hormonally sensitive, stressed to the max, or not sleeping do not pass this point either.*

Mostly c's. You are ready to dive into phase 3. No more dairy, grains, or snacking for you. It's time to optimize your metabolic hormones and get you in gut harmony and fat-burning mode. Here you will experience a lower carb, higher fat, higher fibre diet. The goal here is to maintain your blood sugar while fasting, through using the stores in your body. This phase also challenges you to work with your circadian rhythm and fully optimize your stress, sleep, and gut health.

You will all get to phase 3, and there's no harm in taking your time getting there. This slow and steady approach makes diet changes more achievable, and it will help you to sustain this lifestyle without making it feel like a diet.

Phase 1

In phase 1 we're setting the foundations for the diet plan and working to ramp you up to the ideal plan for you. All recipes are available in **chapter 10**.

You can choose anything from the phase 1 food list, below, that serves as your DIY Meal Map, and swap it for something on the Done-For-You weekly ingredient list. For instance, don't like shrimp? You can swap it out with another Category 1 Protein.

If you are following the Done-For-You meal plans (phase 1 follows the meal map), there's no need to count servings. These have all been calculated for specific macronutrients. If you are staying in phase 1 for an extra week to adjust to the meal system, or if you want to plan your own meals, you can use this list, and the servings, to make your own 5-4-3-2-1 ingredient list.

Phase 1 DIY Meal Map

Phase 1 Food List

Category 1 Proteins
2 servings/day
(5oz. cooked, 6–7oz. raw)
Mollusk (mussels, oysters)
Shrimp
White fish
Turkey
Chicken
Pork
Extra lean/lean beef cuts
Vegan protein powder

Category 2 Proteins
1 serving/day
(5 oz. cooked, 6–7oz. raw)
Salmon
Eggs
Full-fat beef cuts (ideally grass fed or organic)
Lamb

Fruit-based Polyphenols
2 servings/day
(2/3 cup)
Black elderberry (1,400 mg polyphenol)
Blueberry (800mg polyphenol)
Black current (700 mg polyphenol)
Cherry (250 mg polyphenol)
Strawberry, blackberry, raspberry (200 mg polyphenol)

Nut-Based Polyphenols
1 serving/day
(1/4 cup or 1 Tbsp. butter)
Chestnut (500 mg polyphenol)
Hazelnut (250 mg polyphenol)
Pecan (250 mg polyphenol)
GOAL: 2,000 mg (2 g) polyphenols/day

Non-Starchy Vegetables
6 servings/day
(1 cup raw, 1/2 cup cooked)
(Any, most nutrient dense provided here)
Kale
Kohlrabi
Celeriac
Capers
Heart of palm
Mung bean sprouts
Broccoli
Cauliflower
Endive
Zucchini
Spinach, spring greens
Asparagus
Lettuce (all)
Cabbage (all)
Okra
Chard
Mushrooms (Button, white, Portobello, shiitake)
Mustard greens
Arugula
Peppers (all)
Collards
Tomato
Fennel
Radish
Brussels sprouts
Yellow/green beans
Artichokes
Celery
Eggplant
Jicama

Fruits
1 serving/day
Lemon
Lime
Grapefruit
Orange
Apple
1/2 Avocado

Grains
2 servings/day
(Cooked servings)
1/2 cup Rice, white or brown
1/2 cup Any gluten-free grain
1 cup Quinoa
1/2 cup Cooked rice noodles

Starches
1 serving/day
(1 cup cooked)
Pumpkin
Sweet potato
White potato
Winter squash (butternut, kabocha, acorn, assorted)
Turnip
Beet
Carrot
Rutabaga
(1/2 cup, cooked)
Plantain
Cassava
Other tropical starches
(3/4 cup, cooked)
Beans (black, white, pinto, navy, kidney, mung)
Chickpeas
Split peas, black-eyed peas
Lentils
Bean noodles

Fats
1 serving/day
3 Tbsp. Hemp hearts
1/2 cup Full-fat coconut milk
1 Tbsp. Nut or seed butters
1/2 cup Nuts or seeds
1/2 Avocado
3/4 cup Coconut yogurt, unsweetened
1 Tbsp. Oil (avocado, coconut, olive)
8 Olives

Dairy
1 serving/day, maximum
3/4 cup Full-fat yogurt/ kefir
2 oz. Soft cheese
2 oz. Hard cheese
1 Tbsp. Grated cheese
1 Tbsp. Butter/cream

Soluble Fibres
1 serving/day, minimum
2 Tbsp. Chia seed
2 Tbsp. Flax, fresh ground

Fermentable Fibres (raw)
1 serving/day minimum
1 tsp. Chicory root
1 tsp. Jerusalem artichoke
1/2 tsp. Onion
1 tsp. Garlic
1/2 cup Leek
1/2 cup Dandelion greens

Fermented Food
1 serving/day
3/4 cup Coconut yogurt, unsweetened
1 Tbsp. Sauerkraut
1 Tbsp. Kimchi
23 Pickles (lacto-fermented)
1/2 cup Kombucha
2 oz. Tempeh
1 Tbsp. Miso

Beverages
Water (flat or sparkling)
Tea (herbal, green, black)
1 cup Coffee (black, 100 mg polyphenols)
1/2 cup Nut milk or pea milk

Spices
3 servings/day
1 tsp. = 10 mg polyphenol
(All allowed, best polyphenol content herbs follow)
Coriander
Parsley
Basil
Chives
Curry powder
Chili flakes
Chili powder
Oregano
Thyme
Rosemary
Sage
Cinnamon
Nutmeg
Cumin
Ginger
Lemongrass

Condiments/ Sweeteners
Coconut aminos
Vinegars (no sugar added)
Hot sauce (no sugar added)
Lemon
Lime
Stevia, if needed

Supplements
Added Fibre
5 g/day
Acacia gum
Inulin
Psyllium
Glucomannan / Konjac-mannan (PGX)

Phase 1 Done-For-You Meal Plan

	Day 1	Day 2	Day 3	Day 4	Day 5	Day 6	Day 7
Break-fast	Eggs + Roasted Vegetables	Coconut Yogurt Parfait	Vegetable Frittata	Eggs + Roasted Vegetables	Coconut Yogurt Parfait	Eggs + Roasted Vegetables	Coconut Yogurt Parfait
Snack	Cherries + Nuts	Nut + Berry Bar	Cherries + Nuts	Nut + Berry Bars	Cherries + Nuts	Nut + Berry Bars	Nuts
Lunch	Salad with Shrimp	Stuffed Peppers	Salad with Beans	Curry Shrimp Zucchini Noodles	Salad with Eggs	Quinoa + Shrimp Stir-fry	Salad with Beans
Snack	Vegetables + Almond Butter	Guacamole + Veg-etables	Vegetables + Almond Butter	Guacamole + Veg-etables	Vegetables + Almond Butter	Guacamole + Veg-etables	Vegetables + Almond Butter
Dinner	Stuffed Peppers	Vegetable Frittata	Curry Shrimp Zucchini Noodles	Turkey Patties + Roasted Vegetables	Quinoa + Shrimp Stir-fry	Curry Tur-key with Quinoa + Zucchini	Stuffed Portobello Mush-rooms
Fast	12-hour overnight fast	12-hour overnight fast	12-hour overnight fast	12-hour overnight fast	12-hour overnight fast	12-hour overnight fast	12-hour overnight fast

5-4-3-2-1 Weekly Shopping List

Vegetables	Spinach	Portobello mushrooms	Sweet red peppers	Zucchini	Fennel
Polyphenols	Blueberries	Cherries	Coffee	Pantry Nuts (high polyphenol options)	
Fibre	Onion	Garlic	Chia seeds	Hemp hearts	
Proteins	Shrimps	Eggs	Turkey		
Spices	Curry	Oregano	Cinnamon		
Fat	Olive oil	Coconut oil			
Fermented Foods	Sauerkraut	Coconut yogurt			
Fruit	Avocado				
Starch	Black beans				
Grains	Quinoa				
Dairy	Goat cheese				

Phase 2

In phase 2 we see the elimination of all dairy and snacking. This phase also reduces your carbohydrates and increases your fat and fibre.

Phase 2 DIY Meal Map

Phase 2 Food List

Category 1 Proteins
2 servings/day
(5oz. cooked, 6–7oz. raw)
Mollusk (mussels, oysters)
Shrimp
White fish
Turkey
Chicken
Pork
Extra lean/lean beef cuts
Vegan protein powder

Category 2 Proteins
1 serving/day
(5 oz. cooked, 6–7oz. raw)
Salmon
Eggs
Full-fat beef cuts (ideally grass fed or organic)
Lamb

Fruit-based Polyphenols
2 servings/day
(2/3 cup)
Black elderberry (1,400 mg polyphenol)
Blueberry (800 mg polyphenol)
Black current (700 mg polyphenol)
Cherry (250 mg polyphenol)
Strawberry, blackberry, raspberry (200 mg polyphenol)

Nut-Based Polyphenols
1 serving/day
(1/4 cup or 1 Tbsp. butter)
Chestnut (500 mg polyphenol)
Hazelnut (250 mg polyphenol)
Pecan (250 mg polyphenol)
GOAL: 2,000 mg (2 g) polyphenols/day

Non-Starchy Vegetables
7 servings/day
(1 cup raw, 1/2 cup cooked)
(Any, most nutrient dense provided here)
Kale
Kohlrabi
Celeriac
Capers
Heart of palm
Mung bean sprouts
Broccoli
Cauliflower
Endive
Zucchini
Spinach, spring greens
Asparagus
Lettuce (all)
Cabbage (all)
Okra
Chard
Mushrooms (Button, white, portobello, shiitake)
Mustard greens
Arugula
Peppers (all)
Collards
Tomato
Fennel
Radish
Brussels sprouts
Yellow/green beans
Artichokes
Celery
Eggplant
Jicama

Fruits
1 serving/day
Lemon
Lime
Grapefruit
Orange
Apple
1/2 Avocado

Grains
1 serving/day, maximum
(Cooked servings)
1/2 cup Rice, white or brown
1/2 cup Any gluten-free grain
1 cup Quinoa
1/2 cup Cooked rice noodles

Starches
1 serving/day
(1 cup cooked)
Pumpkin
Sweet potato
White Potato
Winter Squash (butternut, kabocha, acorn, assorted)
Turnip
Beet
Carrot
Rutabaga
(1/2 cup, cooked)
Plantain
Cassava
Other tropical starches

Starches. cont.
(3/4 cup, cooked)
Beans (black, white, pinto, navy, kidney, mung)
Chickpeas
Split peas, black-eyed peas
Lentils
Bean noodles

Fats
1 serving/day
3 Tbsp. Hemp hearts
1/2 cup Full-fat coconut milk
1 Tbsp. Nut or seed butters
1/4 cup Nuts or seeds
1/2 Avocado
3/4 cup Coconut yogurt, unsweetened
1 Tbsp. Oil (avocado, coconut, olive)
8 Olives

Soluble Fibres
1 serving/day, minimum
2 Tbsp. Chia seed
2 Tbsp. Flax, fresh ground

Fermentable Fibres (raw)
1 serving/day, minimum
1 tsp. Chicory root
1 tsp. Jerusalem artichoke
1/2 tsp. Onion
1 tsp. Garlic
1/2 cup Leek
1/2 cup Dandelion greens

Fermented Food
1 serving/day
3/4 cup Coconut yogurt, unsweetened
1 Tbsp. Sauerkraut
1 Tbsp. Kimchi
2–3 Pickles (lacto-fermented)
1/2 cup Kombucha
2 oz. Tempeh
1 Tbsp. Miso

Beverages
Water (flat or sparkling)
Tea (herbal, green, black)
1 cup Coffee (black, 100 mg polyphenols)
1/2 cup Nut milk or pea milk

Spices
3 servings/day
1 tsp. = 10 mg polyphenol
(All allowed, best polyphenol content herbs follow)
Coriander
Parsley
Basil
Chives
Curry powder
Chili flakes
Chili powder
Oregano
Thyme
Rosemary
Sage
Cinnamon
Nutmeg
Cumin
Ginger
Lemongrass

Condiments/ Sweeteners
Coconut aminos
Vinegars (no sugar added)
Hot sauce (no sugar added)
Lemon
Lime
Stevia, if needed

Supplements Added Fibre
10 g/day
Acacia gum
Inulin
Psyllium
Glucomannan / Konjac-mannan (PGX)

Phase 2 Done-For-You Meal Plan

	Day 1	Day 2	Day 3	Day 4	Day 5	Day 6	Day 7
Breakfast	Eggs + Vegetables	Very Berry Smoothie	Eggs + Vegetables	Very Berry Smoothie	Eggs + Vegetables	Very Berry Smoothie	Eggs + Leftover Vegetables
Lunch	Salad with Sweet Potatoes and Chicken	Sweet Potatoes + Soft-boiled Eggs	Tempeh Bowl with Avocado Pesto	Spicy Salmon Salad	Salad + Chicken of choice	Salmon Bowl	Salad + Rosemary Chicken
Dinner**	Lemon basil Chicken + Yellow Beans	Chicken Bowl with Avocado Pesto	Salmon + Brussels Sprouts	Chili Pepper Chicken + Vegetables	Spicy Salmon, Rice Noodles + Asparagus	Chili egg bowl	Rosemary Chicken, Rice Noodles and Avocado Pesto
Fast	12-hour overnight fast	12-hour overnight fast	12-hour overnight fast	12-hour overnight fast	14-hour overnight fast	14-hour overnight fast	14-hour overnight fast

**If you are hungry or craving a "dessert," see the recipe for Magic Shell Berry Bowl.

5-4-3-2-1 Weekly Shopping List

Vegetables	Arugula	Asparagus	Yellow beans	White button mushrooms	Brussels sprouts
Polyphenols	Blueberries	Cherries	Coffee	Cocoa	
Fibre	Onion	Garlic	Chia seeds	Hemp hearts	
Proteins	Salmon	Eggs	Chicken		
Spices	Basil	Chili peppers	Rosemary		
Fat	Olive oil	Pantry nuts			
Fermented Foods	Kimchi	Tempeh			
Fruit	Avocado				
Starch	Sweet potato				
Grains	Rice noodles				
Dairy					

Phase 3

In phase 3 you will be testing your boundaries with fasting and be eliminating all grains and dairy. At this point, you will be at the highest fibre, highest fat, and lowest carbohydrate plan.

Phase 3 DIY Meal Map

Phase 3 Food List

Category 1 Proteins
1 serving/ day
(5oz. cooked, 6–7oz, raw)
Mollusk (mussels, oysters)
Shrimp
White fish
Turkey
Chicken
Pork
Extra lean/lean beef cuts
Vegan protein powder

Category 2 Proteins
2 servings/day
(5 oz. cooked, 6–7oz. raw)
Salmon
Eggs
Full-fat beef cuts (ideally grass fed or organic)
Lamb

Fruit-based Polyphenols
1 serving/ day
(2/3 cup)
Black elderberry (1,400 mg polyphenol)
Blueberry (800 mg polyphenol)
Black current (700 mg polyphenol)
Cherry (250 mg polyphenol)
Strawberry, blackberry, raspberry (200 mg polyphenol)

Nut-Based Polyphenols
1 serving/day
(1/4 cup or 1 Tbsp. butter)
Chestnut (500 mg polyphenol)
Hazelnut (250 mg polyphenol)
Pecan (250 mg polyphenol)
GOAL: 2,000 mg (2 g) polyphenols/ day

Non-Starchy Vegetables
8 servings/day
(1 cup raw, 1/2 cup cooked)
(Any, most nutrient dense provided here)
Kale
Kohlrabi
Celeriac
Capers
Heart of palm
Mung bean sprouts
Broccoli
Cauliflower
Endive
Zucchini
Spinach, spring greens
Asparagus
Lettuce (all)
Cabbage (all)
Okra
Chard
Mushrooms (button, white, Portobello, shiitake)
Mustard greens
Arugula
Peppers (all)
Collards
Tomato
Fennel
Radish
Brussels sprouts
Yellow/green beans
Artichokes
Celery
Eggplant
Jicama

Fruits
1 serving/day
Lemon
Lime
Grapefruit
Orange
Apple
1/2 Avocado

Starches
1 serving/day
(1/2 cup cooked)
Pumpkin
Sweet potato
White Potato
Winter Squash (butternut, kabocha, acorn, assorted)
Turnip
Beet
Carrot
Rutabaga

Fats
2 servings/day
3 Tbsp. Hemp hearts
1/2 cup Full-fat coconut milk
1 Tbsp. nut or seed butters
1/4 cup nuts or seeds
1/2 Avocado
3/4 cup Coconut yogurt, unsweetened
1 Tbsp. Oil (avocado, coconut, olive)
8 Olives

Soluble Fibres
1 serving/day,
minimum
2 Tbsp. Chia seed
2 Tbsp. Flax, fresh ground

Fermentable Fibres
(raw)
1 serving/day,
minimum
1 tsp. Chicory root
1 tsp. Jerusalem artichoke
½ tsp. Onion
1 tsp. Garlic
1/2 cup Leek
1/2 cup Dandelion greens

Fermented Food
1 serving/day
3/4 cup Coconut yogurt,
  unsweetened
1 Tbsp. Sauerkraut
1 Tbsp. Kimchi
2–3 Pickles
  (lacto-fermented)
2 oz. Tempeh
1 Tbsp. Miso

Beverages
Water (flat or sparkling)
Tea (herbal, green, black)
1 cup Coffee (black, 100 mg
  polyphenols)
1/2 cup Nut milk or pea
  milk

Spices
3 servings/day
(1 tsp. = 10 mg polyphenol)
All allowed, best polyphe-
  nol content herbs follow
Coriander
Parsley
Basil
Chives
Curry powder
Chili flakes
Chili powder
Oregano
Thyme
Rosemary
Sage
Cinnamon
Nutmeg
Cumin
Ginger
Lemongrass

Condiments/
Sweeteners
Coconut aminos
Vinegars (no sugar added)
Hot sauce, no sugar added
Lemon
Lime
Stevia, if needed

Supplements
Added Fibre
20 g/day
Acacia gum
Inulin
Psyllium
Glucomanna/ Konjac-
  mannan (PGX)

Phase 3 Done-For-You Meal Plan

	Day 1	Day 2	Day 3	Day 4	Day 5	Day 6	Day 7
Breakfast	Avo-Egg Plate	Fasting	Very Berry Smoothie	Avo-Egg Plate	Very Berry Smoothie	Fasting	Avo-Egg Plate
Lunch	Tomato Beef Casserole	Breakfast Smörgås-bord	Tomato Beef Casserole	Asian-inspired Ginger Shrimp + Gut Love Chia Pudding	Avocado Egg Salad	Breakfast Smörgås-bord	Salad with Shrimp
Dinner	Ginger Basil Beef with Vegetables + Gut Love Chia Pudding	Shrimp Spinach Cups + Gut Love Chia Pudding	Asian-inspired Ginger Shrimp	Fasting	Garlic and Thyme Beef with Vegetables + Gut Love Chia Pudding	Garlic Shrimp Over Sautéed Greens with Pumpkin + Gut Love Chia Pudding	Beef + Vegetable Kabobs
Fast	16-hour fast	12-hour fast	12-hour fast	16-hour fast	16-hour fast	12-hour fast	12-hour fast

5-4-3-2-1 Weekly Shopping List

Vegetables	Green peppers	Chard	Spinach	Mung bean sprouts	Tomato
Polyphenols	Blueberry	Strawberry	Coffee	Pantry nuts	
Fibre	Onion	Garlic	Chia seeds	Hemp hearts	
Proteins	Beef	Shrimp	Eggs		
Spices	Basil	Ginger	Thyme		
Fat	Olive oil	Coconut oil			
Fermented Foods	Kimchi	Coconut yogurt			
Fruit	Avocado				
Starch	Pumpkin				
Grains					
Dairy					

Don't forget to access your online resources at **www.sarahwilsonnd.com/loseitbookbonus**. Remember, the pantry lists and master food list for phases 1, 2, and 3 are all here in a printable format. If you don't like a food represented here, you can swap anything from the same categories (i.e., cherries can be swapped for raspberries).

The *Finally* Lose It Food Guide Review

- The keys to success are simplicity and sustainability. The Finally Lose It Program allows you flexibility and accommodates everyone, from the food illiterate to gourmet chef.
- This system uses scientific principles to combine foods in such a way that you will feel full. Foods are nutrient dense, have low insulin demand, and are set up to psychologically serve you based on how you mentally respond to restricted ingredients, treats, and food addiction.
- This system is packed with digestive supportive nutrients, bringing your gut hormones on line, supporting gut bacteria, and lowering inflammation.
- Best of all, this eating plan is freedom focused! You know what to eat, it accounts for lifestyle events, and hey, if you don't have time to eat one morning then you can fast that day. Research tells us working toward weight loss is not just about what we eat and how that food reacts with our body but also when we eat and when we do not eat.

NOTHING CHANGES WITHOUT YOU!

—DANIELLE LAPORTE

9
30-DAY START-UP GUIDE

Congratulations, you have made it through, and now it's time to put everything you've learned into practice! At this point, you may feel excited, apprehensive, and potentially a little overwhelmed. This is natural, since diet and lifestyle changes are something that you've made before and something you likely fear will never work for you. I hope by now you know that this need not be true, but it's important to find the plan that's best for you and your physiology. That's what we're going to do here.

I have asked you to make a lot of changes throughout this book, and I know this isn't easy. I also know that many of you have read through to this point without taking all the actions because you wanted to get an idea of what you were getting yourself into. I have accounted for this! As we go through the first 30 days of this plan, I have laid all out all the homework from each chapter, step by step. My goal is for this chapter to take any overwhelm out of the picture, to help you communicate with your friends, family, and accountability partner what you will be doing at each stage. When people understand what's happening, they know better how to help you—and they want to!

What to Expect When You Are Expecting—Change that Is!

Day 1–10

The start of anything new requires planning, but it also requires conscious effort. At this point in the journey it may not feel natural for you to check in with your daily homework. It will feel like a big effort to plan your meals in a certain way, to clean out your home, and to change your relationship with sleep and stress. I don't say this to scare you, but to be realistic. If you expected this to be a walk in the park, you would probably stop before you even had a chance to start. I will not let that happen! Strap on your big girl panties, and let's push onward.

Day 11–20

On the other side of the first 10 days, things start to feel more possible. At this point, sleep, stress reduction, and new eating patterns are not yet a habit. The system will feel much more comfortable, but it's not quite part of your routine. Cravings for sugar and sweet foods may be reaching their peak by this point. Most patients have said that the first 14 days were the biggest challenge for them, and then the cravings tend to calm down. This is also true of the "low-carb flu," and the grumpiness and fatigue will have decreased by this point. Energy levels and digestion will be getting better every day.

Day 21–30

This is where the magic happens. At this point, you will be feeling really comfortable in the new lifestyle you have set out for yourself; it will feel natural. This is the period when your identity starts to change. You are no longer taking on the identity of someone who is weight loss resistant. You will no longer be feeling powerless in your body, as if your body is working against you. You will likely have hit your stride.

This is the part when people around you start to notice that you're glowing, and you're feeling more confident in your body and more comfortable with the diet and lifestyle changes. It's becoming easier to say no to different foods that you know are counterproductive to your diet, to stress-inducing projects, and to anything that would challenge the positive mindset you have developed for yourself. For the next six to eight weeks, your daily work will continue to cement itself into your identity, your habits, and your lifestyle. You are developing a new baseline. Enjoy the increase in energy, improved digestion, and the weight falling off. Those achievements are yours to keep!

The 30-Day Daily Guide

Day 1

Today is a big day! By now you know that I believe the start of any successful plan lies in organization. That is exactly what today is for. There are three main steps to accomplish today. The first step is to download the workbook from **www.sarahwilsonnd.com/loseitbookbonus** to follow along with the prompts and exercises. The next step is to refer back to your quiz score in **chapter 8** to decide which of the phases to begin with, 1, 2, or 3. Remember, if you have blood sugar regulation issues and if you are currently eating dairy and grains, there's no reason for you to jump into phase 3. That leap would only set you up for failure. (Every seven days you will experiment with moving to the next phase; you will get there!) The third step I have for you today is to eliminate triggers. I want you to take your time on this. Dive into the kitchen and look for ingredients with sugar, artificial sweeteners, high-fructose corn syrup, gluten, hidden dairy, additives or preservatives and trans fats. Before you begin to restock your house, you need to eliminate all the foods that are going to call your name and cause cravings throughout the program.

Day 2

Today you will continue with your planning activities, but now it's time to plan for implementation. One key to success is eliminating decision fatigue, so get out your calendar and look for times in your schedule where you will be able to reread this book and implement the changes. Even if you can carve out 15 to 30 minutes five to seven days per week, that will be a huge win. Enter it right into your calendar and defend this time from other meetings, social events, etc. "Me time" is productive time.

The second goal for today is to find a partner, if you have not already done so. Research shows that you're more likely to succeed if you have an accountability partner, someone who won't accept your excuses and someone who will be on the ride with you. To get more information on how to work with an accountability partner and for an overview of the book and program to share with them go to **www.sarahwilsonnd.com/loseitbookbonus.**

Day 3

Today, review your calendar to look for all the obstacles over the next month. Do you have big meetings or events that you will need to plan for? How are you going to eat to fuel yourself during those times? When will you fit in exercise and self-care time? Other obstacles to plan for include cravings and setbacks. Are you going to have some strong lemon water to help with the cravings? Do you have some pampering bath products to take a relaxing bath? Do you have 90% dark chocolate in the house? What else can you think of to have on hand to curb cravings and ward off setbacks you already know you're prone to?

There's no "on wagon, off wagon" here; it's called life. No need to beat yourself up! When outlining strategies to deal with setbacks, consider in advance how you're going to get back on track. The reality is that you will likely have a time when you get stuck late at work or end up eating something you didn't want to. Write out a list of the setbacks that you will likely experience and what you will do to avoid letting them sabotage your success.

Day 4

Time to start thinking about baseline testing. Appendix A includes a list of medical tests and appendix B lists at-home testing that you can do now so that you can assess your progress. Glucose and insulin testing, inflammation testing, and digestive health testing can be assessed by a naturopathic doctor or medical doctor. In terms of your at-home measurements, it's important to measure your arms, hips, bust, and waist at a minimum. Also track any food sensitivities with the daily symptom log at **www.sarahwilsonnd.com/loseitbookbonus.** Basal body temperature charting will also provide helpful information if you suspect you may have a thyroid issue. (See appendix B.)

People who succeed know their *why*. For instance, if you want to lose weight so that you can feel more confident in your body, play with your kids more, or exercise painlessly, you need to recognize your personal motivation and write it down. We all have a bigger motivation than pounds on a scale, and when you tap into it, that will be the thing that keeps you on track.

Day 5

Woohoo! Today is the day to dive in. You have your meal plan picked, and your shopping list is as simple as can be. Don't forget to pick up the pantry items as well this week, to ensure you have all of those on hand. After shopping is done, get started right away on your meal prep. Need to clean and chop vegetables for the week? Take 30 minutes, which you've scheduled into your calendar, to do so. You can also pre-cook proteins for easy meal assembly.

Day 6

Have you identified your habit-forming style? Are you a moderator or an abstainer? Do you need multiple levels of accountability or do you do better working on your own? This information you can find out in **chapter 7**. I hope it provides you with as much clarity as it provided me!

Given that tomorrow is the start date for your new eating plan, today's the day to have finalized what your week will look like. Are you going to be like me and do major meal prep on Sunday and Thursday? When are you going to fit in your workouts and movement activities, such as walking? Are you going to do your gratitude practice while brewing your morning coffee or before bed? Just scheduling these activities eliminates a lot of decisions you would otherwise have had to make and think about all day. Remember, the goal is to eliminate decision fatigue.

Day 7

Start! Today is Day 1 of the diet changes. You have your meals prepped and ready! Also check in with your accountability partner today to set goals. How do you want to feel? Are you hoping for more energy, less stress, fewer digestive issues? Let your partner know about your goals outside of weight loss. Set a schedule with them.

Are you going to text each other daily or just meet weekly? Find a pace that works for both of you and schedule those calls, texts, or meetings today. The final partner task is to help each other to set non-food rewards. It's easier to rush through life not celebrating your successes than it is to slow down and enjoy them. Getting to the end of this book is a success, prioritizing your health is a success. Set a reward, whatever that looks like to you: a massage, manicure, girl's day out. Hold your partner accountable to the reward, because that positively reinforces the changes you are each making.

Day 8

So many of us eat erratically, but this needs to end. Take some time today to plan mealtimes (including carving out a lunchtime away from your desk). You should also be ensuring that you are fasting at least 12 hours overnight from today onward.

Day 9

Today's challenge is to pucker up to the sour, digestion-stimulating, insulin-reducing power of ACV. Commit to consuming 1–2 tsp. in a little bit of water before each meal. Not only will you see your digestion improve, but this will also improve gut hormone signalling. Remember, if you get a burning or reflux feeling, take the ACV closer to the meal. If symptoms persist, ACV may not be for you.

Day 10

By this time, you should have cut that light at night. The nighttime light inventory (in your workbook **www.sarahwilsonnd.com/loseitbookbonus**) will help you to assess just how many light sources are affecting the quality of your sleep, and thus your degree of inflammation and hormonal balance.

Cutting light at night is not as easy as it may sound. Putting a blue light blocker on your phone or computer (like f.lux) is a great start, but not quite enough. If you are used to sitting in a fully lit living room or watching TV until all hours of the night, this may be a big change for you. Given our urban light pollution, it may be impossible to achieve 100% darkness, but in an effort to limit light stimulation, think of activities you can do instead of the ones you currently engage in before sleep. What about taking a bath, reading a paper book, doing some light yoga or stretching? If you have a lot of light that filters into your bedroom from outside, try blackout curtains or an eye mask, because even this light will affect your sleep hormones and quality of sleep. If you try to reduce light exposure without this planning, you will likely end up twiddling your thumbs and then falling back into old habits because of boredom.

Day 11

Time to work on getting good-quality sleep, which also means enough sleep. If you are not getting enough sleep, you'll need to set a bedtime. Ideally, you would be asleep before 11:00 p.m., but this may be a drastic change for you. Try setting an alarm on your phone to remind you to go to bed just 15 minutes before you normally do now. So, if you generally go to bed at 1:00 a.m., dial that back to 12:45 a.m. for a few nights, and then 12:30 a.m., and continue that pattern, until you have reached 11:00 p.m. If falling to sleep is a challenge, revisit **chapters 2 and 3** for more tips.

Day 12

My experience tells me that today is often when you are feeling overwhelmed, grumpy, tired, and you may even have a headache or flu-like symptoms. This can happen when you are making big changes to your diet, which impacts blood sugar regulation. I often tell people to prepare to grieve today, because you may have a whole range of emotions hit you. If you are feeling down or need more support, today is a great day to text your accountability partner or reach out to your support community to help you to keep on track.

Day 13

Given that these last few days may have been emotionally challenging, I often recommend you look at what other sources of stress may be taking their toll. Stress has such a huge impact on metabolic health and well-being, and as discussed, it can take so many shapes and forms! Take the stress inventory in your workbook today and spend 30 minutes planning how you can begin to remedy some of those stressors. Are you going to ask for more help with commitments? Get testing done for underlying infections? Work on your perception of stress? All of the items you list should have an attached plan to help you get support. Sometimes that support is just journaling your thoughts. Be kind to yourself today and take some action.

Day 14

Stress and self-care are on opposing ends of the same spectrum. Yesterday, you likely thought of some ways to resolve at least some of your stressors, which is a great step toward self-care. What do you do for yourself? Do you take time to be in nature, to cuddle with pets or partners, to read, breathe, stretch? Do you have a hobby that you love but aren't making time for? Plan some specific self-care activities to fill in those parts of your calendar allotted to self-care.

Day 15

One week into the big changes! How are you feeling? Check in with your accountability partner today. What were your wins for the week? Your challenges for the week? Reflect on any mindset challenges and any food triggers you noticed. If you were tracking changes in your journal, reflect back on how you felt and what changes have occurred since?

Day 16

Journaling is a great way to track your progress and reframe your experience. This is especially true of gratitude journaling, because it helps to refill your willpower cup, it helps to change your perspective on the world, and it can truly frame your mindset for the day. Challenge yourself to think of three things that you are grateful for. (Bonus points if one of them is about your body, i.e., I am so grateful for my health, my ability to play with my family, get stronger, and hug my partner.)

Day 17

At this point the plan is likely feeling more doable. You are getting the hang of the routine and feeling more confident with food choices. There may still be a few nagging complaints or things that are not improving the way you wish. If this is the case, go back into the applicable chapter and see if you could benefit from up-levelling with supplements, if you haven't already. For example, if you are still feeling tired and burnt out from the stress of life then an adaptogen formula may be just the thing you need.

Day 18

Avoiding snacks is a critical piece of the metabolic repair and hormone reset that needs to occur in order for you to lose weight and feel healthy in your body. This may feel like it goes against a lot of what you have been told, but in the research, there is no question. Allowing your body time in the fasted state is critical to success in overcoming weight loss resistance. If by this point you are still snacking, or still feeling really hungry between meals, it's imperative to start eating more fat with your meals and drinking more water between them. From this point forward, unless you are really hangry, snacks should be a thing of the past. What to do if you are truly hangry? The best snack choice is a fat option or low-sugar fruit because they do not stimulate insulin to a significant degree and they promote satiety. Nuts and berries or avocado and vegetables will be your best "in a pinch" choices.

Day 19

Whether you know it or not, if you are eating according to the meal plan, you are getting the 2 g of polyphenols needed to start decreasing inflammation, supporting your gut bacteria, and supporting your metabolic hormones. The master foods list offers polyphenol-containing foods. If you don't like one polyphenol source in the meal plan, make sure you are swapping it for another and not just omitting it. These polyphenols are important. So, too, is fibre. If you have not already started, begin slowly increasing your soluble fibre consumption today. Inulin can be added in 1 g increments (see **chapter 5**).

Day 20

It's so easy to get stuck in a rut with what we eat, the types of exercise we do, even the route we take to work. Just as variety is the spice of life, food variety is the key to a diverse range of microbial species in your body for a healthy gut. With increased diversity there is less inflammation, improved immune function, metabolic hormone balance, and even more weight loss! Challenge your mindset today about what you do and don't like. Try a new vegetable, fermented food, or spice that's outside of your comfort zone.

Day 21

You've mastered setting a lunchtime, eating polyphenols, fibre, and even trying new foods. You've come a long way! But are you actually mindful of what you're eating and how much you're chewing your food? As discussed, chewing your food starts the digestion cascade and supports proper gut hormone signalling, which are critical to feeling full and having an appropriate insulin and glucose response to a meal. When was the last time you chewed each bite of food 20, or even 10 times, before you swallowed it? Today, count how many times you chew each bite and see where you land. Ideally, chewing 30 to 40 times per bite will provide maximal benefits to ward off bloating and gas, and also for your waistline.

Day 22

Two weeks down. Can you believe it? Check in with your accountability partner today. What were your wins for the week? Challenges for the week? Reflect on any mindset challenges, and discuss the areas that you're seeing the most progress. The topic of this week's check-in should go beyond food, sleep, stress, and food sensitivities. How is your exercise routine going? Chat with your accountability partner about strategies to incorporate more movement into your day and how to get two to three body weight workouts in.

Day 23

Time for another mindset growth day! It's time to challenge your beliefs about what is possible. At this point you have cut out snacking and are fasting for 12 hours overnight every day, right? Try to fast for 14 hours from today's dinner to tomorrow's breakfast. For example, if you finish dinner at 6:00 p.m., you would not eat breakfast until after 8:00 a.m. During that fasting time, only black coffee, herbal tea, and water with lemon are allowed. These fasts give time to allow your insulin levels to drop, getting you into fat-burning mode. This also helps to begin to reduce the leptin resistance and allow proper turnover of your cells. Don't get stuck in fear and apprehension. You can do this!

Day 24

By now you should be out of the cravings and well on your way to breaking through food triggers and bad habits. If this is not the case, we need to do some more investigation. If you are having cravings, for instance, stop and ask yourself a few questions when they hit.

- Where are you? Is there something about that location that has you driving toward a food?
- What are you just doing? Is there an action such as watching TV or walking to the washroom past the kitchen that has caused the craving onset?
- What time of day is it? Is this a subconscious pattern or a habit? Do you just want a break to get up, stretch, or socialize? This doesn't have to include food.
- What is your emotional state? Are you feeling tired, stressed, overwhelmed, happy, sad?
- Who are you with? Are the actions of certain people leading you to fall back into old patterns? If so, you'll need to be more aware and have stronger boundaries when you're with those people.

Day 25

How is that exercise pact going with your accountability partner? You should have two to three days this week where you have scheduled exercise. As a fun challenge, try to add in 10 to 15 minutes of HIIT today. There are plenty of YouTube videos for this. It will feel challenging if you have not done it before, but you can take it at your own pace. Can't you just feel the insulin resistance decreasing when you do this work out? (It's so challenging that it must be doing something, right?)

Day 26

How's that 14-hour fast going? Did you try it? If you haven't tackled it yet, I'm here to challenge you again. Tonight I want you to embark on your first 16-hour fast. That can be from either 4:00 p.m. to 8:00 a.m., or from 6:00 p.m. to 10:00 a.m., etc. However you can best get it in. A 16-hour fast with an eight-hour eating window has worked wonders for my patients' energy levels, digestion, and weight loss. Once they get over their mental objections, they are often shocked about how easy it is, and how well they feel. However, if you are feeling shaky, nauseous, or have difficulty focusing with a 16-hour fast, you have options. You can go back to 14 hours and slowly increase by 30-minute increments. This should not be done on consecutive days, but two to three times per week. Another option is to have chia seeds with your lemon water to keep you feeling full. You can also play with fat fasting, where you add coconut oil or MCT oil to your coffee and have that for "breakfast." The fat will keep you feeling full and help to support your blood sugar levels without increasing insulin.

Day 27
Now that you're getting comfortable with your new lifestyle changes and feeling better in your body, you may notice your identity starting to shift. This is a great time to keep working on personal development. You are at the start of a journey that's going to require you to see yourself as a healthy, powerful, strong woman who will reach her goals no matter what. If there's a mindset book you want to read, a class or new workout you want to try, now is the time to do it. Keep the momentum of challenging your physical and mental boundaries. This approach helps to ensure you will continue seeing progress in your body as well.

Day 28
Depending on which phase you began with, you may need to plan your meals on your own for the next week. Don't forget to set aside time to do this. It's still a good idea to follow the phase 3 DIY Meal Map, eliminating grains and dairy. This should happen until you have reached your goal weight. Choose recipes you have liked and make a 5-4-3-2-1 food list for yourself to make variations of those meals.

Develop your new baseline further today. What foods are you going to fall back on when you're busy, overwhelmed, and short on time? For me that is vegetables covered with a fat option. Eggs and smoothies are also easy go-to options. The goal is to make eating require very little cognitive draw. This is the key to your ongoing success.

Day 29
Reward yourself! What was the reward you put in place if you kept your promises at day 7? The fact that you made it to the end of this book is a huge achievement! Time to give yourself that non-food reward. Keep up the amazing work!

Day 30
Three weeks eating differently, you've made it so far. Congratulations! Today, check in with your accountability partner. What were your wins for the week? Challenges

for the week? Reflect on any mindset challenges and discuss the areas where you are seeing the most progress. Also review your quizzes with your accountability partner. Have you seen improvements in your sleep, stress, circadian timing, digestion, signs of insulin resistance? Have your arm, bust, waist, and hip measurements decreased? In your accountability meeting today, help each other to meal plan for the next week and set an ongoing schedule for meeting times. Finally, celebrate together!

Bonus Day 1

Plan for ongoing success. Just because the 30-day plan is done doesn't mean that you are. Keep up weekly accountability meetings, continue with your fasting windows, take care of yourself, sleep well, eat well, and continue to work on your perception of stress.

If you want to include public accountability at this stage, that is set up for you. I believe that having multiple levels of accountability is important. Try telling more people about your success or posting about it on social media and having public accountability to help motivate you to continue aiming for your goals. This doesn't work for everyone, but if you are motived to keep on track knowing that you have put it out into the world, it might just be what you need to continue.

To access the success badge for your Facebook, Instagram, or whatever platform your people are on, go to **www.sarahwilsonnd.com/loseitbookbonus.**

Take Action

Be sure to stay connected on social media and tag me with your updates along the way. I want to provide for each of you all the tools and information that I wish I had going through my journey. I look forward to seeing you all succeed!

PART THREE

Recipes for Success

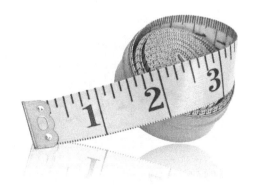

HAPPINESS IS

HOME-MADE.

—ANONYMOUS

10
RECIPES

Eggs + Roasted Vegetables
Yields 1 serving

Ingredients
3 eggs
1/2 bulb fennel
1 cup baby spinach
1 Tbsp. coconut oil
Salt and pepper to taste

Instructions
Eggs
- Heat a skillet over medium heat with ½ Tbsp. coconut oil.
- Fry 3 eggs until cooked.

Roasted Vegetables**
- Heat oven to 300°F.
- Separate fennel bulb into individual leaves.
- Coat fennel with remaining ½ Tbsp. coconut oil.
- Roast for 15 minutes, add spinach, and then roast for 5 extra minutes.

**To prepare vegetables for the week roast 3 servings.

Coconut Yogurt Parfait

Yields 1 serving

Ingredients

3/4 cup coconut yogurt
2/3 cup blueberries
1/3 cup cherries
1 Tbsp. chia seeds
1 Tbsp. hemp hearts
Cinnamon to taste

Instructions

- In a bowl, layer coconut yogurt with blueberries, cherries, ground cinnamon, chia seeds, and hemp hearts.

PHASE 1 BREAKFAST

Vegetable Frittata
Yields 2 servings

Ingredients
4 eggs
2 cups baby spinach
4 oz. portobello mushrooms, chopped
3 Tbsp. coconut milk
2 oz. goat cheese

Instructions
- In a bowl, combine the eggs, spinach, mushrooms, coconut milk, and goat cheese.
- Heat a skillet over medium-low heat and pour mixture into it. Cover and cook on low heat until eggs are cooked through.

Salad with Shrimp

Yields 1 serving

Ingredients
6–7oz. shrimp
2 cups baby spinach
2 Tbsp. sauerkraut
1 Tbsp. hemp hearts
2 Tbsp. olive oil
1 Tbsp. apple cider vinegar
Salt and pepper to taste
1 cup berries of choice

Instructions
- Bring water to a boil in a large pot.
- Place the shrimp in a steamer basket on top of the pot of boiling water.
- Steam shrimp until pink, approximately 5–6 minutes.
- Combine all ingredients in a bowl and add cooked shrimp on top. Berries can be combined in the salad or served on the side

PHASE 1 MAINS

Salad with Beans

Yields 1 serving

Ingredients

3/4 cup black beans, cooked
2 cups baby spinach
2 Tbsp. sauerkraut
1 Tbsp. hemp hearts
2 Tbsp. olive oil
1 Tbsp. apple cider vinegar
1 tsp. Dijon mustard
Salt and pepper to taste
1 cup berries of choice

Instructions

- Combine all ingredients in a bowl and enjoy.
- Berries can be combined in the salad or served on the side

Salad with Eggs

Yields 1 serving

Ingredients

3 eggs

2 cups baby spinach, or other desired vegetable

2 Tbsp. sauerkraut

1 Tbsp. hemp hearts

2 Tbsp. olive oil

1 Tbsp. apple cider vinegar

Salt and pepper to taste

1 cup berries of choice

Instructions

Option 1: Fried Eggs

- Heat a skillet over medium heat with ½ Tbsp. coconut oil.
- Add eggs. Fry eggs until cooked.

OR

Option 2: Hard-Boiled Eggs

- In a small saucepan, cover 3 eggs with cold water until they are submerged at least 1 inch.
- Heat water on high heat until boiled.
- Once boiled, remove pan from heat and cover to let stand for 10 minutes.
- You can either serve the eggs warm or run under cold water to stop the cooking process.

- Combine all ingredients in a bowl and add eggs on top.

PHASE 1 MAINS

Stuffed Peppers

Yields 2 servings

Ingredients

4 large red bell peppers
12–14 oz. ground turkey
1 medium white onion, chopped
2 tsp. garlic, minced
2 cups zucchini, chopped
1/2 cup quinoa, raw
1 cup liquid (water or vegetable stock or bone broth)
2 tsp. dried oregano
2 Tbsp. coconut oil, melted

Instructions

- Place the quinoa and liquid in an uncovered medium saucepan and bring to a boil.
- Once boiling, cover the pan and reduce heat to simmer for 15–20 minutes.
- Fluff with a fork and set aside
- In a medium saucepan, sauté the onion and garlic in coconut oil.
- Add the zucchini and ground turkey and cook until browned.
- Combine dried oregano and quinoa into the ground turkey mixture and cook for an additional 3–5 minutes.
- Preheat oven to 350°F.
- Cut off tops of bell peppers and clean out the seeds. Scoop turkey mixture into peppers and cook for 30 minutes.

Curry Shrimp with Zucchini Noodles

Yields 2 servings

Ingredients

2 large zucchini

1 Tbsp. curry paste

12 oz. shrimp

2 cups raw baby spinach

1 tsp. garlic, minced

1/2 cup white onion, chopped

1 Tbsp. coconut oil

1 can (7 oz.) coconut milk

Instructions

- Using a tool, or spiralizer, make zucchini into noodles. This can also be done with a knife, cutting the zucchini into thin, pasta-sized pieces.
- In a medium saucepan, heat coconut oil and add the onion and garlic and cook until fragrant, then add curry paste.
- Add raw shrimp and the thickened coconut milk from the top of the can into the pan. (If a can of coconut milk has sat, or better yet, been refrigerated, then the thick white cream will separate from the translucent liquid.)
- Cook for 2–3 minutes.
- Add zucchini noodles and spinach and cook until zucchini is at desired tenderness.

PHASE 1 MAINS

Turkey Patties + Roasted Vegetables

Yields 1 serving

Ingredients

1/4 lb ground turkey
1/4 cup quinoa
1/2 cup liquid (water or vegetable stock or bone broth)
1 egg
1 tsp. dried oregano
1 tsp. garlic, minced
1/4 cup white onion, chopped
Salt and pepper to taste
1 Portobello mushroom
1 red bell pepper
1/2 bulb fennel
1 + 1 Tbsp. coconut oil

Instructions

- Place the quinoa and liquid in an uncovered medium saucepan and bring to a boil.
- Once boiling, cover the pan and reduce heat to simmer for 15–20 minutes.
- Fluff with a fork.

Turkey Patties

- Combine turkey, quinoa, egg, oregano, garlic, and white onion.
- Form in the shape of a patty.
- Heat coconut oil in saucepan and cook patty until cooked through (5–7 minutes per side).

Roasted Vegetables

- Heat oven to 300°F.
- Separate fennel bulb into individual leaves.
- Coat fennel, mushroom, and pepper with 1 Tbsp. coconut oil and salt and pepper.
- Roast vegetables for 20 minutes.

Quinoa + Shrimp Stir-fry
Yields 2 servings

Ingredients
1/2 cup quinoa
1 cup liquid (water or vegetable stock or bone broth)
2 Tbsp. coconut oil
1 cup white onion, chopped
8–10 oz. shrimp
1 bell pepper, chopped
4 cups spinach
2-4 Tbsp. coconut aminos, to taste

Instructions
- Place the quinoa and liquid in an uncovered medium saucepan and bring to a boil.
- Once boiling, cover the pan and reduce heat to simmer for 15–20 minutes.
- Fluff with a fork.
- In a medium saucepan heat coconut oil and sauté onion until fragrant. Then add raw shrimp and peppers and cook until shrimp start to turn pink (5–6 minutes).
- Add quinoa, spinach, and coconut aminos and cook for 2–3 more minutes.

Curry Turkey with Quinoa and Zucchini
Yields 1 serving

Ingredients
1/4 cup quinoa

1/2 cup liquid (water or vegetable stock or bone broth)

1 Tbsp. coconut oil

1/4 cup white onion, chopped

1/2 tsp. garlic, minced

1/2 Tbsp. curry paste

6 oz. ground turkey

1/2 can (7 oz.) coconut milk

1 medium zucchini, chopped or spiralized

Instructions
- Place the quinoa and liquid in an uncovered medium saucepan and bring to a boil.
- Once boiling, cover the pan and reduce heat to simmer for 15–20 minutes.
- Fluff with a fork.
- In a medium saucepan heat coconut oil and add the onion and garlic and cook until fragrant then add curry paste.
- Add the ground turkey and cook until browned.
- Add the thickened coconut milk from the top of the can into the pan along with zucchini and cook for 2–3 minutes. Add quinoa.

Stuffed Portobello Mushrooms

Yields 1 serving

Ingredients

1/4 cup quinoa

1/2 cup liquid (water or vegetable stock or bone broth)

2 Portobello mushroom caps

1 tsp. coconut oil

1 tsp. garlic, minced

1/2 cup white onion, chopped

4 oz. ground turkey

1 oz. goat cheese

1 tsp. dried oregano

1/2 medium zucchini, chopped

Instructions

- Place the quinoa and liquid in an uncovered medium saucepan and bring to a boil.
- Once boiling, cover the pan and reduce heat to simmer for 15–20 minutes.
- Fluff with a fork.
- In a medium saucepan heat coconut oil and cook garlic and onion until translucent.
- Add ground turkey and cook until browned.
- Mix cooked turkey, goat cheese, oregano, quinoa, and zucchini and add mixture into both mushroom caps.
- Heat oven to 300°F and cook mushrooms for 20 minutes.

PHASE 1 MAINS

Batch Cooking Quinoa
Yields 4 servings

Ingredients
1 cup quinoa
2 cups liquid* (water or vegetable stock or bone broth)
*Regardless of the amount cooking, the ratio is always 1 cup quinoa to 2 cups liquid.

Instructions
- Place the quinoa and liquid in an uncovered medium saucepan and bring to a boil.
- Once boiling, cover the pan and reduce heat to simmer for 15–20 minutes.
- Fluff with a fork and serve or store.

Nut + Berry Bars
Yields 6 servings

Ingredients
1/2 cup pecans
1/2 cup almonds
1/2 cup cashews
1.5 Tbsp. coconut oil
1/3 cup blueberries
1/3 cup cherries
1/2 tbsp. gelatin
1/4 cup cold water
1/2 tbsp. chia seeds

Instructions
- Soak almonds and cashews for 30 minutes in boiling water.
- Drain almonds and cashews.
- In a food processor combine pecans, almonds, and cashews. Pulse until finely chopped.
- Add melted coconut oil and blend until mixed and slightly sticky.
- Press mixture into a pan and let cool in fridge.
- Bloom gelatin in 1/4 cup of cold water.
- In a saucepan combine fruit and warm on low-medium to bring to a boil. Add bloomed gelatin and chia seeds. Stir and then take off the heat to cool.
- Add cooled fruit mixture on top of nut base and place in the fridge.
- Cut into 6 bars.
- Keep refrigerated.

Guacamole

Yields 1 serving

Ingredients
1/2 medium avocado
1 tsp. lime juice
1 Tbsp. onion, chopped
Salt to taste

Instructions
- In a bowl combine all ingredients until avocado is to your desired texture.
- Serve with vegetables.

Cherries + Nuts

Yields 1 serving

Ingredients
1 cup cherries
15 almonds

Instructions
- Combine in a bowl and enjoy.

Vegetables + Almond Butter
Yields 1 serving

Ingredients
1 Tbsp. almond butter
1/2 bell pepper, cut into strips
1/2 cup fennel, cut into strips

Instructions
- Either spread almond butter over the vegetable strips or use it as a dip.

Eggs + Vegetables
Yields 1 serving**

Ingredients
3 eggs
2 cups vegetable of choice (mushrooms, asparagus, or arugula)
2 Tbsp. chopped onion
1/2 Tbsp. coconut oil
Salt, pepper, and chili flakes to taste
1 cup blueberries

Instructions
- Heat a skillet with coconut oil.
- Add 2 cups of your desired vegetable and cook until softened.
- Remove and set aside.

Option 1: Fried Eggs
- Fry 3 eggs until cooked.

OR

Option 2: Hard-Boiled Eggs
- In a small saucepan cover 3 eggs with cold water until they are submerged at least 1 inch.
- Heat water on high heat until boiled.
- Once boiled, remove pan from heat and cover to let stand for 10 minutes.
- You can either serve the eggs warm or run under cold water to stop the cooking process.
- Combine the cooked egg of your choice with prepared vegetables and add spices. Enjoy blueberries on the side.

**If you like reheated eggs then you can make a two servings at a time.

Very Berry Smoothie
Yields 1 serving

Ingredients
2/3 cup blueberries

1/3 cup cherries

3 Tbsp. hemp hearts

3 Tbsp. chia seeds

1 scoop vegan protein powder

1/2 cup coconut milk (carton)

1 cup greens

Instructions
- Combine all ingredients in a blender and blend until smooth.
- Add more liquid as necessary.

PHASE 2 BREAKFAST

Salad with Sweet Potatoes and Chicken

Yields 1 serving**

Ingredients

6–7oz. chicken breast
2 Tbsp. coconut oil
1 Tbsp. lemon juice
1 tsp. garlic
3 basil leaves, sliced
Salt and pepper to taste
1/3 cup sweet potato slices
2 cups arugula
1 Tbsp. olive oil
1 Tbsp. apple cider vinegar
2 Tbsp. hemp hearts
2 Tbsp. kimchi
1/2 medium avocado

Instructions

- Preheat the oven to 400°F.
- Coat the chicken breast with 1 Tbsp. coconut oil, lemon, basil, garlic, salt, and pepper.
- Coat the sweet potatoes with 1 Tbsp. coconut oil, salt, and pepper.
- Place the chicken and sweet potatoes on a baking sheet and cook for 30–35 minutes.
- Combine the remaining ingredients in a bowl and add cooked sweet potatoes and chicken on top.

**Roast double the chicken and sweet potato for leftovers for dinner and the next day.

Lemon Basil Chicken + Yellow Beans
Yields 1 serving

Ingredients
6–7oz. chicken breast
1 Tbsp. lemon juice
1 tsp. garlic
3 basil leaves, sliced
1 Tbsp. coconut oil
Salt and pepper to taste
1 cup yellow beans
1 cup asparagus
2 Tbsp. kimchi

Instructions
- Preheat oven to 400°F.
- Marinate chicken breast with 1 Tbsp. lemon juice, 1 tsp. garlic, ½ Tbsp. coconut oil, 3 basil leaves, salt, and pepper.
- Coat yellow beans and asparagus with remaining coconut oil, salt, and pepper.
- Place both chicken and vegetables on a baking sheet and bake for 20–25 minutes or until cooked through.

PHASE 2 MAINS

Sweet Potatoes + Soft-Boiled Eggs

Yields 1 serving

Ingredients

1/2 cup sweet potatoes, diced
1 Tbsp. coconut oil
3 eggs
1 tbsp. Dijon mustard
1 tbsp. apple cider vinegar
1 tbsp. olive oil
Salt and pepper to taste
1 cup arugula
1/2 medium avocado

Instructions

- Preheat oven to 400°F.
- Coat diced sweet potato with coconut oil and place on baking dish. Roast sweet potatoes for 30 minutes. (Can also use leftover cooked sweet potatoes.)
- Bring a small pot of water to boil then reduce to a simmer. Add eggs to the pot of water and cook for 5–6 minutes. Remove eggs and run under cold water to stop cooking process. Peel the eggs.
- In a small bowl combine mustard, apple cider vinegar, olive oil, salt, and pepper.
- Combine eggs, sweet potato, arugula, avocado, and dressing in a bowl.

Chicken Bowl with Avocado Pesto*

Yields 1 serving

Ingredients

1/4 cup raw cashews
8 basil leaves, approximately
2 Tbsp. lemon juice
1/2 tsp. garlic
2 Tbsp. hemp hearts
1/2 medium avocado
1 Tbsp. olive oil
1/2 cup water
1/2 tsp. salt
6–7oz. chicken breast, cooked and diced
1/3 cup cooked sweet potato

Instructions

Avocado Pesto

- Combine cashews, basil leaves, lemon juice, garlic, hemp hearts, avocado, olive oil, water, and salt in a food processor/blender.
- Combine until creamy (do not over-blend).

- Combine chicken breast, sweet potato, and avocado pesto.

*Pesto stores well for 2–3 days in the fridge.

Tempeh Bowl with Avocado Pesto*

Yields 1 serving

Ingredients

1/2 cup rice/bean noodles, cooked
4–5 oz. organic tempeh
1 Tbsp. coconut oil
1 Tbsp. coconut aminos
2 Tbsp. hemp hearts
1/4 cup raw cashews
8 basil leaves, approximately
2 Tbsp. lemon juice
1/2 tsp. garlic
1/2 medium avocado
1 Tbsp. olive oil
1/2 cup water
1/2 tsp. salt

Instructions

- Bring 2 cups of water to a boil and add rice/bean noodles.
- Let the noodles cook for 5–10 minutes, or until tender.
- In a medium frying pan, heat coconut oil and coconut aminos.
- Slice tempeh either into cubes or strips.
- Fry tempeh pieces in coconut oil and coconut aminos until browned.

Avocado Pesto

- Combine cashews, basil leaves, lemon juice, garlic, avocado, olive oil, water and salt in a food processor/blender.
- Combine until creamy (do not over-blend).

- Combine all ingredients in a bowl and enjoy.

*Pesto stores well for 2–3 days in the fridge.

Salmon + Brussels Sprouts
Yields 1 serving**

Ingredients
6–7 oz. salmon filet
1 Tbsp. coconut oil
1/2 tsp. clove garlic, minced
Salt and pepper to taste
2 cups Brussels sprouts
2 Tbsp. lemon juice
1/2 cup white onion, chopped

Instructions
- Preheat oven to 400°F.
- Place the salmon filet in a piece of tinfoil. Coat with ½ Tbsp. coconut oil, garlic, salt, pepper, and 1 Tbsp. lemon juice.
- In a separate bowl coat Brussels sprouts with ½ Tbsp. coconut oil, 1 Tbsp. lemon juice, and white onion.
- Place tinfoil packet and Brussels sprouts on baking sheet and cook for 12–15 minutes. Remove salmon.
- Continue to cook Brussels sprouts for an additional 10 minutes.

**Double the salmon recipe for lunch the next day.

PHASE 2 MAINS

Lemon Salmon Salad

Yields 1 serving

Ingredients

6–7oz. salmon filet
1/2 Tbsp. coconut oil
1/2 tsp. garlic
1 Tbsp. lemon juice
4 cups arugula
2 Tbsp. olive oil
2 Tbsp. apple cider vinegar
3 Tbsp. hemp hearts
4 Tbsp. kimchi
1/2 medium avocado
Salt and pepper to taste

Instructions

- Preheat oven to 400°F.
- Place the salmon filet in a piece of tinfoil. Coat with ½ Tbsp. coconut oil, garlic, salt, pepper, and 1 Tbsp. lemon juice.
- Cook salmon for 12–15 minutes.
- Combine the remaining ingredients in a bowl and add cooked salmon on top.

Chili Pepper Chicken + Vegetables
Yields 1 serving**

Ingredients
6–7oz. chicken breast
2 Tbsp. coconut oil
1 tsp. dried chili flakes
1/2 tsp. garlic, minced
1/2 cup sweet potatoes, diced
1/2 cup white onion, chopped
3/4 cup white button mushrooms

Instructions
- Heat oven to 400°F.
- Coat chicken breast with chili flakes, 1 Tbsp. coconut oil, and garlic.
- Coat sweet potatoes, onion, and mushrooms with 1 Tbsp. coconut oil.
- Place chicken in centre of baking tray and surround with vegetable mixture.
- Cook for 30–35 minutes or until cooked through.

**Double chicken for leftovers for lunch tomorrow or alternatively prepare rosemary chicken.

PHASE 2 MAINS

Salad + Chicken
Yields 1 serving

Ingredients
6–7 oz. chicken breast
1 Tbsp. coconut oil
1 tsp. rosemary, chopped
Salt and pepper to taste
2 cups arugula
1 Tbsp. apple cider vinegar
2 Tbsp. hemp hearts
2 Tbsp. kimchi
1/2 medium avocado

Instructions
- Preheat the oven to 400°F.
- Coat the chicken breast with 1 Tbsp. coconut oil, rosemary, salt and pepper. (You can also use leftover chili chicken.)
- Combine the remaining ingredients in a bowl and add cooked chicken on top.

Spicy Salmon, Rice Noodles + Asparagus
Yields 1 serving + left over salmon

Ingredients
2x 6–7oz salmon filet
3 Tbsp. coconut oil
1/2 tsp. garlic, minced
2 Tbsp. Dijon mustard
1 Tbsp. coconut aminos
10 asparagus stalks
Salt and pepper to taste
1/2 cup rice/bean noodles, cooked
1 Tbsp. kimchi

Instructions
- Preheat oven to 400°F.
- Place the salmon filet in a piece of tinfoil. Coat with 2 Tbsp. coconut oil, garlic, Dijon mustard, and coconut aminos.
- In bowl coat asparagus stalks with 1 Tbsp. of coconut oil, salt, and pepper.
- Place salmon and asparagus stalks on baking tray and cook for 12–15 minutes.
- Place asparagus and one salmon filet on top of cooked rice/bean noodles and mix with kimchi.

Salmon Bowl

Yields 1 serving

Ingredients
4-5oz. salmon filet, leftover
1/2 medium avocado
1 Tbsp. olive oil
1 Tbsp. lemon juice
2 cups arugula
10 stalks of asparagus
1 Tbsp. hemp hearts
Salt and pepper to taste

Instructions
• Combine all ingredients in a bowl and mix.

Chili Egg Bowl

Yields 1 serving

Ingredients

1 Tbsp. coconut oil

1/3 cup sweet potato, chopped

1 cup yellow beans, chopped

10 stalks of asparagus

1/2 cup mushrooms

1/4 tsp. chili flakes

Salt and pepper to taste

3 large eggs, boiled

1 Tbsp. Dijon mustard

Instructions

- Add coconut oil to a skillet and add sweet potato. Sauté for 10 minutes over medium heat.
- Add beans, asparagus, mushrooms, chili, and salt and pepper to taste. Cover and cook for 10 minutes.
- Add boiled eggs and Dijon mustard.
- Combine in a bowl and mix.

PHASE 2 MAINS

PHASE 2 MAINS

Chicken, Rice Noodles, + Avocado Pesto*
Yields 1 serving

Instructions
4–5 oz. leftover chicken breast, cooked, chopped
1/2 cup rice/bean noodles, cooked
1/4 cup raw cashews
8 basil leaves, approximately
2 Tbsp. lemon juice
1 clove garlic
1/2 medium avocado
1 Tbsp. olive oil
1/2 cup water
1/2 tsp. salt

Instructions
- Combine cooked, chopped chicken with avocado pesto and cooked rice/bean noodles.

Avocado Pesto
- Combine cashews, basil leaves, lemon juice, garlic, avocado, olive oil, water and salt in a food processor/blender.
- Combine until creamy (do not over-blend).

*Pesto stores well for 2-3 days in the fridge.

Magic shell berry bowl

Yields 1 serving

Ingredients

1/2 cup frozen blueberries

1/2 cup frozen cherries

1 Tbsp. coconut oil

1/2 Tbsp. cocoa powder

Pinch of salt

Stevia to taste

Instructions

- Add frozen berries to a bowl and let thaw 10–15 minutes.
- In a separate bowl mix coconut oil, cocoa, salt, and stevia. Melt if needed so that it is a liquid consistency.
- Drizzle melted cocoa mixture over partially frozen berries, let harden. Crack and enjoy!

PHASE 2 SNACKS

Fasting

Instructions
1 cup black coffee or tea

OR
1 cup water
1/2 lemon, juiced
2 Tbsp. chia seeds

Avo-Egg Plate

Yields 1 serving

Ingredients

3 eggs

1/2 Tbsp. coconut oil

1/2 medium avocado, diced

1 Tbsp. kimchi

1/2 cup blueberries

1/2 cup strawberries

Instructions

Eggs:

- Heat a skillet with ½ Tbsp. coconut oil.
- Fry 3 eggs until cooked.*
- On a plate top eggs with diced avocado and kimchi. Serve with a side of berries.

*You can hard-boil the eggs instead if preferred.

PHASE 3 BREAKFAST

Very Berry Smoothie

Yields 1 serving

Ingredients

2/3 cup blueberries
1/3 cup strawberries
3 Tbsp. hemp hearts
3 Tbsp. chia seeds
1 scoop vegan protein powder
1/2 cup coconut milk (carton)
1 cup greens

Instructions

- Combine all ingredients in a blender and blend until smooth.
- Add more liquid as necessary.

Tomato Beef Casserole

Yields 3 servings

Ingredients

1 Tbsp. coconut oil
1 lb ground beef
1 cup white onion, chopped
1 garlic clove, minced
1 cup green pepper, chopped
3 cups Swiss chard, shredded
3 cups diced tomatoes
1 tsp. salt
1 tsp. pepper

Instructions

- In a large saucepan heat coconut oil on medium-high heat.
- Add white onion and garlic. Cook until translucent, approximately 5 minutes.
- Add ground beef and cook until browned, approximately 10-15 minutes.
- Add green peppers, Swiss chard, tomatoes, salt, and pepper and mix.
- Reduce heat to a simmer and let cook for 60 minutes.

Ginger Basil Beef with Vegetables
Yields 1 serving

Ingredients
1/2 cup pumpkin
2 Tbsp. coconut oil
1/3 lb ground beef
1/4 tsp. fresh ginger, grated
1/2 tsp. garlic, minced
1 tsp. fresh basil, chopped
2 cups baby spinach
1/4 cup coconut milk (can)
Salt and pepper to taste

Instructions
- Heat oven to 300°F.
- On a baking sheet coat pumpkin with 1 Tbsp. coconut oil, salt, and pepper.
- Bake pumpkin for 30 minutes or until tender.
- While the pumpkin bakes, heat 1 Tbsp. coconut oil in a medium saucepan.
- Add ground beef, ginger, basil, garlic, and cook for 10–15 minutes. Add baby spinach and coconut milk and cook for another 5–10 minutes.

Breakfast Smörgåsbord

Yields 1 serving

Ingredients

3/4 cup coconut yogurt
1 cup blueberries
1/2 cup strawberries
1 Tbsp. hemp hearts
1 Tbsp. chia seeds
1 tsp. coconut oil
2 eggs
1/2 cup Swiss chard
Salt and pepper to taste
1/2 medium avocado

Instructions

- Combine coconut yogurt, berries, hemp hearts, and chia seeds in a bowl.
- Heat coconut oil in a skillet. Add eggs and Swiss chard, scramble. Add salt and pepper.
- Serve with a side of avocado.

PHASE 3 MAINS

Shrimp Spinach Cups

Yields 1 serving

Ingredients
6 oz. shrimp
1 Tbsp. coconut oil
1/4 cup raw cashews, chopped
1/2 Tbsp. coconut aminos
1 cup bean sprouts
10 large spinach leaves
2 Tbsp. kimchi

Instructions
- Chop shrimp and sauté in coconut oil along with the chopped cashew for 5 minutes. Add coconut aminos and bean sprouts, and sauté for another 2–3 minutes.
- Divide shrimp mixture and serve in a spinach leaf cup (2 leaves together), along with kimchi.

Asian-Inspired Ginger Shrimp
Yields 2 servings

Ingredients
12 oz. shrimp
2 Tbsp. coconut oil
1/2 cup white onion, chopped
2 tsp. garlic, minced
1/2 tsp. ginger, grated
2 cups Swiss chard
2 Tbsp. almond butter
1 Tbsp. coconut aminos

Instructions
- Bring water to a boil in a large pot.
- Place the shrimp in a steamer basket on top of the pot of boiling water and steam shrimp until pink, about 5–6 minutes.
- In a small saucepan heat coconut oil over medium heat with white onion, garlic, ginger and Swiss chard. Cook for about 10 minutes until Swiss chard is wilted. Add almond butter and coconut aminos.
- Add shrimp and heat for another 1–2 minutes.

Avocado Egg Salad
Yields 1 serving

Ingredients
3 eggs
1/2 medium avocado
2 cups spinach
1/2 cup mung bean sprouts
1/4 cup tomato, chopped
2 tbsp. hemp hearts
2 tbsp. sauerkraut
1 tbsp. olive oil
2 tbsp. apple cider vinegar
Salt and pepper to taste

Instructions
- Eggs: Bring a small pot of water to boil then reduce to simmer. Add eggs to the pot of water and cook for 5-6 minutes. Remove eggs and run under cold water to stop cooking process. Peel the eggs.
- Mash eggs with avocado and combine with vegetables, hemp hearts, and sauerkraut. Add olive oil and vinegar dressing and enjoy.

Garlic and Thyme Beef with Vegetables
Yields 1 serving

Ingredients
5 oz. beef tenderloin
2 Tbsp. coconut oil
1 tsp. dried thyme
1 tsp. garlic, minced
1/4 cup white onion, chopped
1/2 green pepper, chopped
2 cups Swiss chard

Instructions
- Heat oven to 350°F.
- Coat the beef tenderloin with 1 Tbsp. coconut oil, ½ the garlic, and thyme.
- Place tenderloin into a roasting pan and cook uncovered for 30–40 minutes.
- In the meantime, heat 1 Tbsp. coconut oil in a small saucepan. Add white onion and ½ tsp. garlic cook until transparent. Sauté green pepper and Swiss chard until desired doneness.
- Once tenderloin is cooked to desired redness, cover in tinfoil and let it sit for 10–15 minutes.
- Once slightly cooled, slice to desired thickness and serve with vegetables.

PHASE 3 MAINS

Garlic Shrimp over Sautéed Greens with Pumpkin

Yields 1 serving

Ingredients
1/2 cup pumpkin, chopped
2 Tbsp. coconut oil
Salt and pepper to taste
6–7oz. shrimp
1/2 tsp. garlic, minced
1/4 cup white onion, chopped
2 cups Swiss chard

Instructions
- Heat oven to 300°F.
- On a baking sheet coat pumpkin with 1 Tbsp. coconut oil, salt, and pepper. Bake pumpkin in the oven for 30 minutes or until tender.
- Bring water to a boil in a large pot.
- Place the shrimp in a steamer basket on top of the pot of boiling water and steam shrimp until pink.
- In a medium saucepan heat 1 Tbsp. coconut oil and add garlic.
- Sautee the onion and Swiss chard.
- Add the steamed shrimp to the saucepan and cook for another 2–3 minutes.

Salad with Shrimp
Yields 1 serving

Ingredients
6–7oz. shrimp
2 cups spinach
1/2 cup mung bean sprouts
1/2 cup tomato, chopped
1/2 medium avocado
2 Tbsp. hemp hearts
2 Tbsp. kimchi
2 Tbsp. olive oil
2 Tbsp. apple cider vinegar
1 tsp. mustard
1/2 Tbsp. coconut aminos
Salt and pepper to taste

Instructions
- Bring water to a boil in a large pot.
- Place the shrimp in a steamer basket on top of the pot of boiling water and steam shrimp until pink, approximately 5–6 minutes.
- Combine the rest of the ingredients in a bowl and top with steamed shrimp.

Beef and Vegetable Kabobs

Yields 1 serving

Ingredients

5–6 oz. beef steak

2 Tbsp. avocado oil

1/2 tsp. dried thyme

1 tsp. garlic, minced

1 white onion, peeled and cut into chunks for skewering

1 green pepper, cut into squares

Instructions

- Cut the beef into cubed pieces.
- Combine avocado oil, thyme, and garlic.
- Marinade the beef for 20 minutes (or longer if you have time).
- Using wooden skewers alternate the beef, onion, and pepper.
- Heat barbecue to 400°F.
- Cook beef until desired redness, usually 5–6 minutes.

Gut Love Chia Pudding

Yields 4 servings

Ingredients

1 cup chia seeds
3+ cups of coconut or almond milk (carton), dilute to desired consistency
1 tsp. vanilla Stevia to taste
40 g inulin powder

Chocolate Chia
For a chocolate variation add 2 Tbsp. of cocoa powder to the chia mix before soaking.

Chai Chia
For a chai variation, add 1/4 tsp. cinnamon.
Omit 1 cup of nut milk and add strong brewed chai tea.

Instructions

- Place the chia seeds, nut milk, vanilla, stevia, and inulin in a bowl and stir well so there are no clumps and all the chia seeds are coated in milk.
- Let this sit at room temperature for 20–30 minutes, or cover and refrigerate.

This pudding will keep well in the refrigerator for days.

APPENDIX A

Laboratory Investigations and Optimal Ranges for Metabolic Health

This is an exhaustive list of tests that can be ordered by your medical doctor or naturopathic doctor. Although suggested reference ranges are provided on laboratory reports, "normal" is not always "optimal." Therefore, I have included my preferred ranges below.

Metabolic Health Laboratory testing	Optimal Range (SI units)	Optimal Range (Conventional units)
Fasting insulin	<50 pmol/L	<7 units/mL
Fasting glucose	4.8–5.5 mmol/L	80–95 mg/dL
2-hr post challenge insulin	<220 pmol/L	<30 units/mL
2-hr post challenge glucose	<6.0 mmol/L	90–140 mg/dL
HbA1c	<5.0%	<5.0%
Erythrocyte sedimentation rate (ESR)	<5 mm/hr	<5 mm/hr
High-sensitivity c-reactive protein (hs-CRP)	<1.0 mg/L	< 1.0 mg/L
Thyroid stimulating hormone (TSH)	1.0–2.5 mIU/L	1.0–2.5 mIU/L
Free T3	Variable, depending on the person	Variable, depending on the person
Free T4	Units vary: top 1/2 normal range	Units vary: top 1/2 normal range
Total Cholesterol	3.9–5.7 mmol/L	150–220 mg/dL
LDL	2.6–3.4 mmol/L	100–130 mg/dL
HDL	1.3–1.8 mmol/L	50–70 mg/dL
Triglycerides	<1.7 mmol/L	<70 mg/dL
Vitamin D	100–150 nmol/L	40–60 ng/mL
Ferritin	40–90 mcg/L	40–90 ng/mL
Iron	9–18 umol/L	50–100 ug/dL

Note: Optimal ranges are different than those considered diagnostic. These levels are considered desirable for optimal health.

APPENDIX B
AT-HOME TESTING

Blood Glucose Monitoring

At-home blood glucose monitors are now widely available at pharmacies and online retailers. This provides an opportunity to get a lot of information about your health and your body's response to food. This is especially true if you do not have access to a naturopathic doctor or medical doctor who is willing to support you with lab work.

Just as a blood draw for fasting glucose would be done, you can measure fasting glucose levels with your at-home monitor. Upon waking, clean a finger and prick with a clean lancet. Wipe the first drop of blood away and then use the second drop of blood to sample. Fasting glucose levels should be the same as fasting glucose levels listed above. Then you would do the same two hours after finishing a meal.

I recommend doing this test before starting the program, with a usual meal. Then repeat during phase 1, phase 2, and phase 3 meals, once per week to assess your tolerance for carbohydrates.

If your blood sugar is spiking after eating sweet potato but not fruit, then this can provide information about which foods will keep you metabolically healthy.

Although there is no at-home test on the market for insulin, blood glucose testing can give at least some insight into your body's response to a food. Keep in mind, though, glucose does not cause weight gain. If your levels are normal that's great! But it may require twice the normal insulin release to keep those levels within range. That is why finding a provider who can test insulin levels will provide the most insight.

Basal Body Temperature Charting

Basal body temperature charting, or BBT charting, provides information about your metabolic capacity, more specifically about your female sex hormones and thyroid. Although I did not discuss thyroid function extensively in this book, as it's a complex topic all its own, I want to make mention of it.

Your thyroid is a gland in the front of your neck that releases hormones that control your metabolic rate. When your thyroid is humming along it supports your metabolic rate and this can be estimated by your body temperature on waking.

This is important to understand before starting the protocol and as you make diet changes. Some people are unable to tolerate a lower carbohydrate diet in the long term. These people will witness a consistently lower body temperature after making diet changes. The key to understand here is consistence, meaning greater than 3 weeks of persistently low temperatures.

It's important to note that your body temperature is controlled by many factors including sleep, stress, alcohol, and ovulation. That said, if your temperature is consistently falling below the range provided, it may be important to get blood work done to assess thyroid function. If it drops consistently low only after making diet changes, and you are feeling tired, cold, have brain fog and slower bowels, it may be time to try to change your macronutrients again to see if this reverses itself.

How to BBT Chart

Buy a basal body temperature thermometer from a local pharmacy or online. These are often available in the family planning section. The difference between a BBT thermometer and a conventional thermometer is the extra decimal place (i.e., 36.12 vs 36.1°C). This extra decimal place is important for the accuracy of this exercise.

Have your thermometer on your bedside table and measure your temperature each morning before sitting up, standing, or exerting yourself in any way. Record this temperature on paper or in a period tracking app.

If you find that you get an afternoon energy slump between 2:00 p.m. and 4:00 p.m., you can also measure your temperature at that time. Temperature levels should be higher during this time than in the morning. Although not a basal temperature, it can still provide useful information as to what could be contributing to that energy fall.

As your BBT cycles with your female sex hormones, you will need to take your temperature consistently for 30–60 days to assess progress and accuracy. If your temperature is consistently lower than 36.5°C (or 97.7°F) upon waking, even after a good night's sleep, then check in with a medical provider.

REFERENCES

1. Eckel-Mahan, K. & Sassone-Corsi, P. Metabolism and the circadian clock converge. *Physiol. Rev.* **93**, 107–135 (2013).

2. Horne, J. A. & Ostberg, O. A self-assessment questionnaire to determine morningness-eveningness in human circadian rhythms. *Int. J. Chronobiol.* **4**, 97–110 (1976).

3. Sarabia, J. A., Rol, M. A., Mendiola, P. & Madrid, J. A. Circadian rhythm of wrist temperature in normal-living subjects. *Physiol. Behav.* **95**, 570–580 (2008).

4. Challet, E. Keeping circadian time with hormones. *Diabetes, Obes. Metab.* **17**, 76–83 (2015).

5. Garaulet, M. & Gómez-Abellán, P. Timing of food intake and obesity: A novel association. *Physiol. Behav.* **134**, 44–50 (2014).

6. Bandín, C., Martinez-Nicolas, A., Ordovás, J. M., Madrid, J. A. & Garaulet, M. Circadian rhythmicity as a predictor of weight-loss effectiveness. *Int. J. Obes.* **38**, 1083–1088 (2014).

7. Scully, C. G. et al. Skin surface temperature rhythms as potential circadian biomarkers for personalized chronotherapeutics in cancer patients. *Interface Focus* **1**, (2010).

8. Reid, K. J. et al. Timing and Intensity of Light Correlate with Body Weight in Adults. *PLoS One* **9**, e92251 (2014).

9. Ross, K. M., Graham Thomas, J. & Wing, R. R. Successful weight loss maintenance associated with morning chronotype and better sleep quality. *J. Behav. Med.* **39**, 465–471 (2016).

10. Oike, H., Oishi, K. & Kobori, M. Nutrients, Clock Genes, and Chrononutrition. *Curr. Nutr. Rep.* **3**, 204–212 (2014).

11. Knutson, K. L., Spiegel, K., Penev, P. & Van Cauter, E. The metabolic consequences of sleep deprivation. *Sleep Med. Rev.* **11**, 163–178 (2007).

12. Colten, H. R., Altevogt, B. M. & Research, I. of M. (US) C. on S. M. and. Sleep Physiology. (2006).

13. Kim, T. W., Jeong, J.-H. & Hong, S.-C. The impact of sleep and circadian disturbance on hormones and metabolism. *Int. J. Endocrinol.* **2015**, 591729 (2015).

14. Besedovsky, L., Lange, T. & Born, J. Sleep and immune function. *Pflugers Arch.* **463**, 121–137 (2012).

15. Hurtado-Alvarado, G. et al. Sleep loss as a factor to induce cellular and molecular inflammatory variations. *Clin. Dev. Immunol.* **2013**, 801341 (2013).

16. Bollinger, T. et al. Sleep-dependent activity of T cells and regulatory T cells. *Clin. Exp. Immunol.* **155**, 231–238 (2009).

17. Walecka-Kapica, E. *et al.* The effect of melatonin supplementation on the quality of sleep and weight status in postmenopausal women. *Prz. menopauzalny = Menopause Rev.* **13,** 334–338 (2014).

18. Baker, F. C. & Driver, H. S. Circadian rhythms, sleep, and the menstrual cycle. *Sleep Med.* **8,** 613–622 (2007).

19. Knutson, K. L. & Van Cauter, E. Associations between sleep loss and increased risk of obesity and diabetes. *Ann. N. Y. Acad. Sci.* **1129,** 287–304 (2008).

20. Taheri, S., Lin, L., Austin, D., Young, T. & Mignot, E. Short sleep duration is associated with reduced leptin, elevated ghrelin, and increased body mass index. *PLoS Med.* **1,** e62 (2004).

21. von Loeffelholz, C. *The Role of Non-exercise Activity Thermogenesis in Human Obesity. Endotext* (MDText.com, Inc., 2000).

22. Novak, C. M. & Levine, J. A. Central Neural and Endocrine Mechanisms of Non-Exercise Activity Thermogenesis and Their Potential Impact on Obesity. *J. Neuroendocrinol.* **19,** 923–940 (2007).

23. Chase, J. E. & Gidal, B. E. Melatonin: therapeutic use in sleep disorders. *Ann. Pharmacother.* **31,** 1218–1226 (1997).

24. Held, K. *et al.* Oral Mg(2+) supplementation reverses age-related neuroendocrine and sleep EEG changes in humans. *Pharmacopsychiatry* **35,** 135–143 (2002).

25. Nielsen, F. H., Johnson, L. K. & Zeng, H. Magnesium supplementation improves indicators of low magnesium status and inflammatory stress in adults older than 51 years with poor quality sleep. *Magnes. Res.* **23,** 158–168 (2010).

26. Geer, E. B., Islam, J. & Buettner, C. Mechanisms of glucocorticoid-induced insulin resistance: focus on adipose tissue function and lipid metabolism. *Endocrinol. Metab. Clin. North Am.* **43,** 75–102 (2014).

27. Samra, J. S. *et al.* Effects of Physiological Hypercortisolemia on the Regulation of Lipolysis in Subcutaneous Adipose Tissue [1]. *J. Clin. Endocrinol. Metab.* **83,** 626–631 (1998).

28. Djurhuus, C. B. *et al.* Additive effects of cortisol and growth hormone on regional and systemic lipolysis in humans. *AJP Endocrinol. Metab.* **286,** 488E–494 (2003).

29. Adam, T. C. *et al.* Cortisol Is Negatively Associated with Insulin Sensitivity in Overweight Latino Youth. *J. Clin. Endocrinol. Metab.* **95,** 4729–4735 (2010).

30. Savastano, S. *et al.* Role of dehydroepiandrosterone sulfate levels on body composition after laparoscopic adjustable gastric banding in pre-menopausal morbidly obese women. *J. Endocrinol. Invest.* **28,** 509–515 (2005).

31. Levy, A. *et al.* Co-sensitivity to the incentive properties of palatable food and cocaine in rats; implications for co-morbid addictions. *Addict. Biol.* **18,** 763–773 (2013).

32. Adam, T. C. & Epel, E. S. Stress, eating and the reward system. *Physiol. Behav.* **91,** 449–458 (2007).

33. for Disease Control, U. . C. & Center for Environmental Health, N. Second National Report on Biochemical Indicators of Diet and Nutrition in the U.S. Population. (2012).

34. Morita, E. *et al.* Psychological effects of forest environments on healthy adults: Shinrin-yoku (forest-air bathing, walking) as a possible method of stress reduction. *Public Health* **121,** 54–63 (2007).

35. Park, B.-J. *et al.* Physiological effects of Shinrin-yoku (taking in the atmosphere of the forest)--using salivary cortisol and cerebral activity as indicators. *J. Physiol. Anthropol.* **26,** 123–128 (2007).

36. Jankowski, M., Broderick, T. L. & Gutkowska, J. Oxytocin and cardioprotection in diabetes and obesity. *BMC Endocr. Disord.* **16,** 34 (2016).

37. Horn, S. R., Charney, D. S. & Feder, A. Understanding resilience: New approaches for preventing and treating PTSD. *Exp. Neurol.* **284,** 119–132 (2016).

38. Pascoe, M. C. & Bauer, I. E. A systematic review of randomised control trials on the effects of yoga on stress measures and mood. *J. Psychiatr. Res.* **68,** 270–282 (2015).

39. Lim, S.-A. & Cheong, K.-J. Regular Yoga Practice Improves Antioxidant Status, Immune Function, and Stress Hormone Releases in Young Healthy People: A Randomized, Double-Blind, Controlled Pilot Study. *J. Altern. Complement. Med.* **21,** 530–538 (2015).

40. Nieuwenhuizen, A. G. & Rutters, F. The hypothalamic-pituitary-adrenal-axis in the regulation of energy balance. *Physiol. Behav.* **94,** 169–177 (2008).

41. Sharma, A. K., Basu, I. & Singh, S. Efficacy and Safety of Ashwagandha Root Extract in Subclinical Hypothyroid Patients: A Double-Blind, Randomized Placebo-Controlled Trial. *J. Altern. Complement. Med.* acm.2017.0183 (2017). doi:10.1089/acm.2017.0183

42. Jacquet, A., Grolleau, A., Jove, J., Lassalle, R. & Moore, N. Burnout: evaluation of the efficacy and tolerability of TARGET 1(R) for professional fatigue syndrome (burnout). *J. Int. Med. Res.* **43,** 54–66 (2015).

43. Talbott, S. M., Talbott, J. A. & Pugh, M. Effect of Magnolia officinalis and Phellodendron amurense (Relora®) on cortisol and psychological mood state in moderately stressed subjects. *J. Int. Soc. Sports Nutr.* **10,** 37 (2013).

44. Kalman, D. S. *et al.* Effect of a proprietary Magnolia and Phellodendronextract on stress levels in healthy women: a pilot, double-blind, placebo-controlled clinical trial. *Nutr. J.* **7,** 11 (2008).

45. Appleton, J. Lavender Oil for Anxiety and Depression. *Nat. Med. J.* **4,** (2012).

46. Morita, H. *et al.* Effect of royal jelly ingestion for six months on healthy volunteers. *Nutr. J.* **11,** 77 (2012).

47. Chiu, H.-F. *et al.* Hypocholesterolemic efficacy of royal jelly in healthy mild hypercholesterolemic adults. *Pharm. Biol.* **55,** 497–502 (2017).

48. Münstedt, K., Bargello, M. & Hauenschild, A. Royal Jelly Reduces the Serum Glucose Levels in Healthy Subjects. *J. Med. Food* **12,** 1170–1172 (2009).

49. Starks, M. A., Starks, S. L., Kingsley, M., Purpura, M. & Jäger, R. The effects of phosphatidylserine on endocrine response to moderate intensity exercise. *J. Int. Soc. Sports Nutr.* **5,** 11 (2008).

50. Hellhammer, J. et al. Effects of Soy Lecithin Phosphatidic Acid and Phosphatidylserine Complex (PAS) on the Endocrine and Psychological Responses to Mental Stress. *Stress* **7**, 119–126 (2004).

51. Benton, D., Donohoe, R. T., Sillance, B. & Nabb, S. The influence of phosphatidylserine supplementation on mood and heart rate when faced with an acute stressor. *Nutr. Neurosci.* **4**, 169–178 (2001).

52. De Silva, A. & Bloom, S. R. Gut Hormones and Appetite Control: A Focus on PYY and GLP-1 as Therapeutic Targets in Obesity. *Gut Liver* **6**, 10–20 (2012).

53. Katschinski, M. Nutritional implications of cephalic phase gastrointestinal responses. *Appetite* **34**, 189–196 (2000).

54. McLaughlin, J. T. & McKie, S. Human brain responses to gastrointestinal nutrients and gut hormones. *Curr. Opin. Pharmacol.* **31**, 8–12 (2016).

55. Xiong, S.-W. et al. Effect of Modified Roux-en-Y Gastric Bypass Surgery on GLP-1, GIP in Patients with Type 2 Diabetes Mellitus. *Gastroenterol. Res. Pract.* **2015**, 625196 (2015).

56. Burcelin, R. The incretins: a link between nutrients and well-being. *Br. J. Nutr.* **93 Suppl 1**, S147-156 (2005).

57. Campbell, J. & Drucker, D. Pharmacology, Physiology, and Mechanisms of Incretin Hormone Action. *Cell Metab.* **17**, 819–837 (2013).

58. Larder, R. & O'Rahilly, S. Shedding pounds after going under the knife: Guts over glory?why diets fail. *Nat. Med.* **18**, 666–667 (2012).

59. Rose, C., Parker, A., Jefferson, B. & Cartmell, E. The Characterization of Feces and Urine: A Review of the Literature to Inform Advanced Treatment Technology. *Crit. Rev. Environ. Sci. Technol.* **45**, 1827–1879 (2015).

60. Harakeh, S. M. et al. Gut Microbiota: A Contributing Factor to Obesity. *Front. Cell. Infect. Microbiol.* **6**, 95 (2016).

61. Boutagy, N. E., McMillan, R. P., Frisard, M. I. & Hulver, M. W. Metabolic endotoxemia with obesity: Is it real and is it relevant? *Biochimie* **124**, 11–20 (2016).

62. Cani, P. D. et al. Metabolic Endotoxemia Initiates Obesity and Insulin Resistance. *Diabetes* **56**, (2007).

63. Neves, A. L., Coelho, J., Couto, L., Leite-Moreira, A. & Roncon-Albuquerque, R. Metabolic endotoxemia: a molecular link between obesity and cardiovascular risk. *J. Mol. Endocrinol.* **51**, R51-64 (2013).

64. Butaye, P., Devriese, L. A. & Haesebrouck, F. Antimicrobial growth promoters used in animal feed: effects of less well known antibiotics on gram-positive bacteria. *Clin. Microbiol. Rev.* **16**, 175–188 (2003).

65. Cox, L. M. & Blaser, M. J. Antibiotics in early life and obesity. *Nat. Rev. Endocrinol.* **11**, 182–190 (2015).

66. Jakubowicz, D. et al. Fasting Until Noon Triggers Increased Postprandial Hyperglycemia and Impaired Insulin Response After Lunch and Dinner in Individuals With Type 2 Diabetes: A Randomized Clinical Trial. *Diabetes Care* **38**, 1820–1826 (2015).

67. Belinova, L. *et al.* The effect of meal frequency in a reduced-energy regimen on the gastrointestinal and appetite hormones in patients with type 2 diabetes: A randomised crossover study. *PLoS One* **12**, e0174820 (2017).

68. Yoo, J. Y. & Kim, S. S. Probiotics and Prebiotics: Present Status and Future Perspectives on Metabolic Disorders. (2016). doi:10.3390/nu8030173

69. Guess, N. D., Dornhorst, A., Oliver, N. & Frost, G. S. A Randomised Crossover Trial: The Effect of Inulin on Glucose Homeostasis in Subtypes of Prediabetes. *Ann. Nutr. Metab.* **68**, 26–34 (2015).

70. Dehghan, P., Pourghassem Gargari, B. & Asghari Jafar-abadi, M. Oligofructose-enriched inulin improves some inflammatory markers and metabolic endotoxemia in women with type 2 diabetes mellitus: A randomized controlled clinical trial. *Nutrition* **30**, 418–423 (2014).

71. Dewulf, E. M. *et al.* Insight into the prebiotic concept: lessons from an exploratory, double blind intervention study with inulin-type fructans in obese women. *Gut* **62**, 1112–1121 (2013).

72. Babiker, R. *et al.* Effects of Gum Arabic ingestion on body mass index and body fat percentage in healthy adult females: two-arm randomized, placebo controlled, double-blind trial. *Nutr. J.* **11**, 111 (2012).

73. Dehghan, P., Pourghassem Gargari, B. & Asghari Jafar-abadi, M. Oligofructose-enriched inulin improves some inflammatory markers and metabolic endotoxemia in women with type 2 diabetes mellitus: A randomized controlled clinical trial. *Nutrition* **30**, 418–423 (2014).

74. Karimi, P. *et al.* The Therapeutic Potential of Resistant Starch in Modulation of Insulin Resistance, Endotoxemia, Oxidative Stress and Antioxidant Biomarkers in Women with Type 2 Diabetes: A Randomized Controlled Clinical Trial. *Ann. Nutr. Metab.* **68**, 85–93 (2015).

75. Sood, N., Baker, W. L. & Coleman, C. I. Effect of glucomannan on plasma lipid and glucose concentrations, body weight, and blood pressure: systematic review and meta-analysis. *Am. J. Clin. Nutr.* **88**, 1167–1175 (2008).

76. Geurts, L., Neyrinck, A. M., Delzenne, N. M., Knauf, C. & Cani, P. D. Gut microbiota controls adipose tissue expansion, gut barrier and glucose metabolism: novel insights into molecular targets and interventions using prebiotics. *Benef. Microbes* **5**, 3–17 (2014).

77. Panickar, K. S. Effects of dietary polyphenols on neuroregulatory factors and pathways that mediate food intake and energy regulation in obesity. *Mol. Nutr. Food Res.* **57**, 34–47 (2013).

78. Solayman, M. *et al.* Polyphenols: Potential Future Arsenals in the Treatment of Diabetes. *Curr. Pharm. Des.* **22**, 549–565 (2016).

79. Kim, Y., Keogh, J. B. & Clifton, P. M. Polyphenols and Glycemic Control. *Nutrients* **8**, (2016).

80. Pérez-Jiménez, J., Neveu, V., Vos, F. & Scalbert, A. Identification of the 100 richest dietary sources of polyphenols: an application of the Phenol-Explorer database. *Eur. J. Clin. Nutr.* **64**, S112–S120 (2010).

81. Engen, P. A., Green, S. J., Voigt, R. M., Forsyth, C. B. & Keshavarzian, A. The Gastrointestinal Microbiome: Alcohol Effects on the Composition of Intestinal Microbiota. *Alcohol Res.* **37,** 223–236 (2015).

82. Cicero, A. F. G. & Colletti, A. Role of phytochemicals in the management of metabolic syndrome. *Phytomedicine* **23,** 1134–1144 (2016).

83. Xu, J., Liu, X., Pan, W. & Zou, D. Berberine protects against diet-induced obesity through regulating metabolic endotoxemia and gut hormone levels. *Mol. Med. Rep.* **15,** 2765–2787 (2017).

84. Lyte, J. M., Gabler, N. K. & Hollis, J. H. Postprandial serum endotoxin in healthy humans is modulated by dietary fat in a randomized, controlled, cross-over study. *Lipids Health Dis.* **15,** 186 (2016).

85. Holt, S. H., Miller, J. C. & Petocz, P. An insulin index of foods: the insulin demand generated by 1000-kJ portions of common foods. *Am. J. Clin. Nutr.* **66,** 1264–1276 (1997).

86. Bell, K. J. *et al.* Estimating insulin demand for protein-containing foods using the food insulin index. *Eur. J. Clin. Nutr.* **68,** 1055–1059 (2014).

87. Beck-Nielsen, H., Pedersen, O. & Lindskov, H. O. Impaired cellular insulin binding and insulin sensitivity induced by high-fructose feeding in normal subjects. *Am. J. Clin. Nutr.* **33,** 273–278 (1980).

88. Stanhope, K. L. *et al.* Consuming fructose-sweetened, not glucose-sweetened, beverages increases visceral adiposity and lipids and decreases insulin sensitivity in overweight/obese humans. *J. Clin. Invest.* **119,** 1322–1334 (2009).

89. Higgins, S., Fedewa, M. V., Hathaway, E. D., Schmidt, M. D. & Evans, E. M. Sprint interval and moderate-intensity cycling training differentially affect adiposity and aerobic capacity in overweight young-adult women. *Appl. Physiol. Nutr. Metab.* **41,** 1177–1183 (2016).

90. Steckling, F. *et al.* High Intensity Interval Training Reduces the Levels of Serum Inflammatory Cytokine on Women with Metabolic Syndrome. *Exp. Clin. Endocrinol. Diabetes* **124,** 597–601 (2016).

91. Gillen, J. B. *et al.* Twelve Weeks of Sprint Interval Training Improves Indices of Cardiometabolic Health Similar to Traditional Endurance Training despite a Five-Fold Lower Exercise Volume and Time Commitment. *PLoS One* **11,** e0154075 (2016).

92. Little, J. P., Jung, M. E., Wright, A. E., Wright, W. & Manders, R. J. F. Effects of high-intensity interval exercise versus continuous moderate-intensity exercise on postprandial glycemic control assessed by continuous glucose monitoring in obese adults. *Appl. Physiol. Nutr. Metab.* **39,** 835–841 (2014).

93. Garbossa, S. G. & Folli, F. Vitamin D, sub-inflammation and insulin resistance. A window on a potential role for the interaction between bone and glucose metabolism. *Rev. Endocr. Metab. Disord.* **18,** 243–258 (2017).

94. Wang, X., Chang, X., Zhu, Y., Wang, H. & Sun, K. Metabolically Obese Individuals of Normal Weight Have a High Risk of 25-Hydroxyvitamin D Deficiency. *Am. J. Med. Sci.* **352,** 360–367 (2016).

95. Abbott, K. A., Burrows, T. L., Thota, R. N., Acharya, S. & Garg, M. L. Do -3
     PUFAs affect insulin resistance in a sex-specific manner? A systematic review and
     meta-analysis of randomized controlled trials. *Am. J. Clin. Nutr.* **104,** 1470–1484
     (2016).

96. Johnston, C. S., Kim, C. M. & Buller, A. J. Vinegar Improves Insulin Sensitivity
     to a High-Carbohydrate Meal in Subjects With Insulin Resistance or Type 2
     Diabetes. *Diabetes Care* **27,** 281 LP-282 (2003).

97. Ostman, E., Granfeldt, Y., Persson, L. & Bjorck, I. Vinegar supplementation low-
     ers glucose and insulin responses and increases satiety after a bread meal in
     healthy subjects. *Eur. J. Clin. Nutr.* **59,** 983–988 (2005).

98. White, A. M. & Johnston, C. S. Vinegar Ingestion at Bedtime Moderates Waking
     Glucose Concentrations in Adults With Well-Controlled Type 2 Diabetes.
     Diabetes Care **30,** 2814 LP-2815 (2007).

99. *Social Neuroscience: Biological Approaches to Social Psychology.* (Routledge, 2016).

100. Kelly, J. D. Your Best Life: Breaking the Cycle: The Power of Gratitude. *Clin.
     Orthop. Relat. Res.* **474,** 2594–2597 (2016).

101. DuBois, C. M., Millstein, R. A., Celano, C. M., Wexler, D. J. & Huffman, J. C.
     Feasibility and Acceptability of a Positive Psychological Intervention for Patients
     With Type 2 Diabetes. *Prim. Care Companion CNS Disord.* **18,** (2016).

102. Holt, S. H., Miller, J. C., Petocz, P. & Farmakalidis, E. A satiety index of common
     foods. *Eur. J. Clin. Nutr.* **49,** 675–690 (1995).